Nutrition and Oral Health

Gerry McKenna

Editor

Nutrition and Oral Health

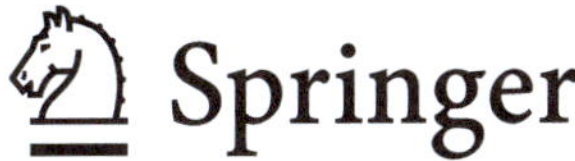
Springer

Editor
Gerry McKenna
Centre for Public Health
School of Medicine
Dentistry and Biomedical Sciences
Queen's University Belfast
Belfast
United Kingdom

ISBN 978-3-030-80528-9   ISBN 978-3-030-80526-5   (eBook)
https://doi.org/10.1007/978-3-030-80526-5

This Springer imprint is published by the registered company Springer Nature Switzerland AG
The registered company address is: Gewerbestrasse 11, 6330 Cham, Switzerland

Contents

Introduction

Gerry McKenna

Abstract

Good-quality nutrition is extremely important for everyone through their life course as it drives growth and development in children and helps prevent many systemic diseases in adults and malnutrition in older adults. Whilst a series of complex and interconnected factors play a role in dietary intake and nutrition, oral health is an important consideration, particularly the maintenance and retention of natural teeth as people age. This book will detail the relationship between oral health and nutrition, with a focus on the extremes of age, by referencing relevant scientific literature and discussing guidance produced by government and public health bodies.

A healthy diet is essential for good health and nutrition at all stages of life as it protects against many chronic non-communicable diseases. Eating a variety of foods and consuming less salt, sugars and saturated and industrially produced trans fats are essential for a healthy diet. A healthy diet comprises a combination of different foods including staples like cereals or starchy tubers; legumes; fruits and vegetables; and proteins from animal sources [1].

Unfortunately, diets are suboptimal for health amongst both adults and children globally. In high-income societies in particular, there is an overconsumption of foods high in fat, salt and sugar, coupled with inadequate intakes of fibre, wholegrains, fruits and vegetables, and fish. Linked to poor-quality dietary intake, there has also been a significant increase in levels of obesity, with rates tripling in adults in the United Kingdom in the past 20 years [2]. This has led to an increase in obesity-related comorbidities such as type 2 diabetes, cardiovascular disease and certain cancers. There is consensus amongst experts that long-term, effective diet and lifestyle changes are needed to improve population health, alongside substantial changes to social and environmental drivers within the food system [3]. Significant advances have been made in the field of behavioural science in the past decade, with a greater shared understanding of the important strategies and techniques which can be used in the design of interventions to change dietary behaviour.

Amongst the complex factors which influence diet and nutritional status, oral health plays an important role. The presence of natural teeth is essential to facilitate mastication, directly impacting nutritional status. The importance of good oral health to facilitate dietary intake is observed most acutely at the extremes of age. Children and adolescents have high nutritional requirements

G. McKenna (✉)
Centre for Public Health, School of Medicine, Dentistry and Biomedical Sciences, Queen's University Belfast, Belfast, United Kingdom
e-mail: g.mckenna@qub.ac.uk

© Springer Nature Switzerland AG 2021
G. McKenna (ed.), *Nutrition and Oral Health*, https://doi.org/10.1007/978-3-030-80526-5_1

relative to their size in order to meet demands for growth, development and physical activity. Dietary habits established in childhood will influence systemic health across the life course. Good nutritional status and good oral health are interconnected; good nutrition is essential for optimal growth, development and maintenance of all tissues and organs in the body, including the oral cavity. Poor or inadequate dietary habits can negatively impact oral health, whilst oral health issues can lead to inadequate nutritional intakes impacting on weight gain and growth.

In older adults, losing natural teeth can impact on masticatory function making it more difficult to chew certain types of foods, such as raw vegetables and fruits as well as some sources of protein. This often leads to a change in food consumption, with an increase in the intake of softer, more processed foods which are low in nutrients and fibre but high in calories [4]. This is particularly apparent in edentate older adults who often present with a higher prevalence of malnutrition or undernutrition compared to their partially dentate counterparts [5]. Changes in oral epidemiology clearly chart the emergence of this partially dentate older population as patients retain natural teeth into old age. This represents a major public dental health success but also a significant challenge as clinicians are now charged with preventing and managing chronic dental diseases for these patients. Dietary intake has now become an important risk factor for chronic dental diseases such as root caries in older adults particularly where high levels of refined carbohydrates are consumed [6].

This book is designed to describe the interrelationship between oral health and nutrition. Given this broad subject, we have focused on children and older adults where clear evidence is available to describe these relationships. For oral health clinicians it is hoped that this information can help inform preventative and operative treatment planning which includes an appreciation of nutrition and dietary intake. For other healthcare professionals it is hoped that this book will help to reinforce the importance of good oral health for management and prevention of systemic diseases particularly in relation to nutrition. To summarise we should remember the position statement of the American Dietetic Association who stated:

"Nutrition and oral health are inextricably linked. Poor oral health can affect an individual's ability to eat certain nutritious foods while poor nutrition can increase an individual's risk of poor oral health including periodontal disease and tooth loss" [7].

References

1. Healthy Diet Fact Sheet. World Health Organization: https://www.who.int/initiatives/behealthy/healthy-diet
2. Scheelbeek PFD, Cornelsen L, Marteau TM, Jebb SA, Smith RD. Potential impact on prevalence of obesity in the UK of a 20% price increase in high sugar snacks: modelling study. BMJ. 2019;366:l4786. https://doi.org/10.1136/bmj.l4786.
3. McGinnis JM, Williams-Russo P, Knickman JR. The case for more active policy attention to health promotion. New York: Health Affairs; 2002. https://doi.org/10.1377/hlthaff.21.2.78.
4. Schimmel M, Genton L, McKenna G. Masticatory function and nutritional status : considerations for an ageing population. In: Oral rehabilitation for compromised and elderly patients. Cham: Springer; 2018. https://doi.org/10.1007/978-3-319-76129-9_6.
5. Watson S, McGowan L, McCrum L-A, et al. The impact of dental status on perceived ability to eat certain foods and nutrient intakes in older adults: Cross-sectional analysis of the UK National Diet and Nutrition Survey 2008–2014. Int J Behav Nutr Phys Act. 2019;16(1):43. https://doi.org/10.1186/s12966-019-0803-8.
6. Hayes M, Da Mata C, Cole M, McKenna G, Burke F, Allen PF. Risk indicators associated with root caries in independently living older adults. J Dent. 2016;51:8–14. https://doi.org/10.1016/j.jdent.2016.05.006.
7. Touger-Decker R, Mobley C. Position of the academy of nutrition and dietetics: oral health and nutrition. J Acad Nutr Diet. 2013;113(5):693–701. https://doi.org/10.1016/j.jand.2013.03.001.

Nutritional Considerations in Children

Ciaran G. Forde, Michelle C. McKinley, Jayne V. Woodside, and Anne P. Nugent

Abstract

Children and adolescents have high nutritional requirements relative to their size in order to meet demands for growth, development and physical activity. Dietary patterns and habits established early in life will influence health in the short and longer term. Good nutritional status and good oral health are interconnected; good nutrition is essential for optimal growth, development and maintenance of all tissues and organs in the body, including the oral cav- ity. Poor or inadequate dietary habits can neg- atively impact oral health whilst oral health problems including dental caries, infection, dental erosion and soft-tissue lesions can result in inadequate nutrition which may impact weight gain and ultimately growth. This chapter describes the development of the oral anatomy and feeding skills, the impact of solid food introduction and the importance of nutrition for growth and development.

C. G. Forde
Sensory Science and Eating Behaviour, Division of Human Nutrition and Health, Wageningen University, Wageningen, The Netherlands

M. C. McKinley · J. V. Woodside
The Institute for Global Food Security, School of Biological Sciences, Queen's University Belfast, Belfast, United Kingdom

Centre for Public Health, School of Medicine, Dentistry and Biomedical Sciences, Queen's University Belfast, Belfast, United Kingdom

A. P. Nugent (✉)
The Institute for Global Food Security, School of Biological Sciences, Queen's University Belfast, Belfast, United Kingdom

Institute of Food and Health, University College Dublin, Dublin, Ireland
e-mail: a.nugent@qub.ac.uk

2.1 Growth and Development in Children

The stages of early life may be broadly defined as infancy, preschool years, childhood and adoles- cence. Each of these periods has its own energy and nutrient requirements reflecting specific rates of growth and development. The first year of life (infancy) is characterised as a time of extraordi- nary growth and development, with rates of growth slowing over the next 10 years or so until adolescence and thereafter accelerating again during puberty until adulthood. Growth height typically ceases at around 16 years of age for girls and 18 years for boys but with muscle and bone development continuing for both sexes until well into adulthood. Unique patterns of cellular and somatic growth occur for all physiological systems throughout this time including the skel- etal system and associated dentition. Matching quantity and quality of food intake with physical activity patterns and growth during this time is important to avoid rapid or delayed weight gain, where rapid weight gain above reference standards has been consistently associated with increased obesity risk [1–3].

2.2 Development of Oral Anatomy, Feeding Skills and Transition to Childhood Eating Behaviours

2.2.1 Importance of the Development of Mastication to Infant Nutrition and Growth

The development of oral anatomy and the feeding skills required to masticate and swallow foods safely and efficiently are central to supporting infants attain the energy and nutrients required for growth during weaning and early childhood. It is often assumed that learning to chew is simply the emergence of an infant's first teeth. However, this process involves many complex and dynamic changes to oral anatomy and neuromuscular coordination during the development of the fine motor skills required to support mastication and swallowing. Mastication is required to prepare food for digestion and ensure that it is safe to swallow, and attaining these skills broadens the dietary diversity available to the developing infant [4]. The oral phase of digestion plays a key role in breaking food particles down to enhance enzymatic hydrolysis of nutrients and increases later absorption during digestion [5, 6]. In addition, the ability to sense foods during consumption has a positive impact on cephalic phase responses and necessary learning that links energy intake and eating behaviours to the development of satiation and post-ingestive feelings of satiety [7]. Whereas the development of oral anatomy progresses naturally with increased chronological age, the evolution of the feeding skills required for mastication and safe swallowing are not innate, but rather have to be learned during a complex period of dynamic change in oral volume, denti-

tion and fine motor skills. During this period the infant will transition from parent-dependent milk feeding to child-led independent feeding on complementary foods with complex sensory properties and textures. This transition marks the move to higher energy intakes from a much wider variety of foods and can only be achieved by learning to evolve from suckling to sucking, biting, munching and eventually chewing more challenging food textures [8, 9]. The ability to successfully masticate and process foods is necessary to attain the nutrition required for successful growth and development.

2.2.2 Development of Oral Anatomy and Mastication During Infancy and Early Childhood

Newborn infants are born with an oral anatomy that is optimised to support suckling during breast and/or bottle feeding. However within the first 24 months of life, their oral anatomy undergoes enormous changes in the transition to a toddler's oral cavity that has the requisite volume, dentition and muscle coordination to masticate and swallow complex textures. The distinct components of the infant's oral anatomy concurrently develop during this transition, including changes to soft tissue, bone and teeth and neuromuscular skills necessary to coordinate efficient mastication and swallowing. The lips, tongue, soft tissues and cheeks are initially filled with fat deposits to tightly position the tongue at the centre of the oral cavity, reducing the risk of swallowing the tongue and choking whilst also creating the necessary seal for suction during suckling. The tongue and lips initially function to latch and secure the infant during suckling and for tongue propulsion, to remove unwanted materials from the oral cavity and reduce the risk of choking. During the transition to complementary foods, the tongue and lips elongate and are reshaped, and their movement becomes much more coordinated to provide the infant with the dexterity required to move food between occlusal surfaces for crushing and to gather food fragments during bolus formation. As the infant grows, their oral volume will increase as fat deposits in the cheeks disappear and jaw bones elongate to create the necessary space for additional tongue movement and later tooth eruption. These soft tissues play an important role in holding and positioning foods between occlusal surfaces to grind and pulverise food and support agglomeration of fragmented pieces for bolus formation [10, 11].

The increase in oral volume is necessary for the eruption of infant dentition and is supported by an elongation in the upper (maxilla) and lower (mandible) jaw bones, and an extension of the palate. A staged emergence of teeth occurs concurrently with the development of oral skills for the manipulation of increasingly harder and more complex food textures, with each additional tooth offering new functionality to the developing infant. The successful development of mastication has a mutually beneficial role of creating access to new nutrient sources in the diet, whilst the act of mastication also helps to extend palate length and create space for the healthy emergence of more teeth, whilst increasing the alignment of occlusal surfaces.

The third key component of oral development is the elongation, strengthening and coordination of the muscles required to elevate (masseters and temporalis muscles) and depress (digastric muscle) the jaw during biting and chewing [12]. Muscle activity in the splanchnocranium and orofacial muscles is regulated by oro-motor central pattern generators and the associated neural networks. These generators control primary behaviours such as respiration, sucking, licking and mastication and optimise over time with experience-dependent mechanisms to promote safe swallowing [13]. There are also reported differences between breast- and bottle-fed children, as those that are breast-fed for up to 12 months receive greater stimulation to orofacial muscles and have been reported to have greater masticatory function [14]. The apparent simplicity of chewing and swallowing belies an enormous complexity, with coordination among at least 26 pairs of muscles and 5 cranial nerve systems [15, 16]. Importantly, these processes are not innate but are learned through highly adaptive and experience-dependent feedback, gathered through repeated exposure to a wide variety of different solid and semi-solid food textures [17]. The synchrony required to co-ordinate muscle contraction and relaxation develops steadily from 12 to 48 months and varies widely across children [12].

Whereas the initial diet is liquid and consumed in a supine position, by 5–6 months most infants can sit upright and are ready to receive complementary foods that are consumed with a spoon or cup. An improvement in muscle coordination and fine motor skills enables the infant to remove semi-solid purees from a spoon using a sucking action with their lips [8]. For more complex semi-solid foods infants rely on 'munching' wherein they process the bolus using vertical movements of the tongue [18]. Over time as feeding skills begin to mature, munching becomes more frequent than sucking and with the emergence of the first incisors the infant learns to bite for the first time. The rate of development of muscle thickness and coordination is dependent on the experience with different textures and there is a mutually beneficial relationship between the development of oral anatomy and processing skills and exposure to new texture challenges [18]. Mastication patterns vary greatly between foods, and the infant learns to adjust this systematically during a chewing sequence based on feedback from the bolus during deformation [13]. During this period the infant also learns to adapt their bite force to the food textures served and quickly recognises textures that cannot be manipulated and chewed, and should be rejected [19].

There is a marked improvement in chewing efficiency between 6 and 10 months with a decrease in chews *per* bite and chew duration during this period. From 10 months onwards, munching becomes more frequent than sucking, progressing alongside a gradual shift to more textured foods [17]. Whereas munching is characterised by vertical jaw movements, chewing involves a more lateral and diagonal movement which continues to develop between 1 and 2 years until eventually the child is capable of the rotary chewing movement associated with efficient mastication [20]. Bite force increases with age during the transition from primary to permanent dentition and with the maturation of the masticatory muscles, and this supports the consumption of harder and more complex food textures encountered in the adult diet [21]. The available bite force is substantially greater in magnitude than that required for normal mastication, and is therefore a poor measure of masticatory efficiency or function, instead reflecting the masticatory muscle thickness and the health of the periodontal tissues [22–25]. Food texture acceptance develops longitudinally, alongside oral development, with only one study to date profiling longitudinal changes in texture preferences over time among a group of infants between 6 and 18 months [26]. The findings highlight a time-dependent evolution of texture acceptance that tracks against oral development, from accepting sticky textures (8 months) to harder foods (12 months) and raw pieces (18 months). Children are capable of chewing by 8 months and this is well established by 10 months, coinciding with shifts to accept more challenging textures that rely on a wider range of oral manipulations and processing skills [26].

Whereas the approach to complementary food introduction and its timing are widely agreed to be of high importance for oral development and later food acceptance, research is still required to better align the functional capacity of the infant with suitable texture challenges that will stimulate oral development [26]. The development of oral anatomy continues alongside the progression to harder and more complex food textures, and with experience the number of chewing cycles decreases from 2 to 4 years as mastication becomes more efficient in reducing and hydrating food structures to form a swallowable bolus [11, 21]. However as this relationship is mutually beneficial, if children do not transition to harder and more challenging food textures at the right phase of their development, this can lead to delayed oral development, feeding difficulties and problems with food texture acceptance in later childhood.

2.2.3 The Impact of Food Texture Introduction on Oral Anatomy and Eating Behaviour

Exposing young children to a wide variety of food textures promotes experiential learning and texture acceptance, and encourages the child to adapt their chewing behaviour and muscle activity to a more diverse set of textural challenges. This is central to the development of oral anatomy and processing skills but also promotes acceptance of a wider variety of nutrient-dense foods with diverse textures that often pose more of a mastication challenge, such as fruits and vegetables [27]. Importantly, there is a high variability in the development of oral processing abilities among children of the same age which leads to wide variability in texture preferences, acceptance and dietary intakes. Children can have poor masticatory efficiency due to sustained consumption of softer foods into later childhood, which delays their exposure to more challenging textures that support healthy tooth eruption and alignment and the development of feeding skills [28]. The timing and quality of food texture introduction have been shown to have an impact on oral development, with research suggesting a sensitive period for introducing more textured foods following the disappearance of tongue protrusion at around 4 months, to promote maximum texture acceptance later in childhood [29]. Late introduction of lumpy and solid textures may promote feeding difficulties, with a greater proportion of children reporting problems when textures were introduced later than 10 months, compared to those who received textures before 6 months [30]. This 'sensitive period' would mean introducing solid textures earlier than is currently recommended by the World Health Organization (WHO), which proposes that mothers should exclusively breastfeed for the first 6 months with no additional food or water source. However, it may be that earlier introduction of solids is important to support infants in learning to process and accept more complex food textures before 6 months. The positive impact of introducing more challenging textures during this sensitive period is not well known, but it has been suggested to offer an important window to promote later food-texture acceptance and access to a broader dietary variety [31]. Recent findings highlight that puree foods with soft lumps are widely accepted by infants <6 months which may have the added benefit of stimulating more tongue movements and improving oral dexterity [21, 26]. In addition to tongue dexterity, differences in children's chew rate are largely dependent on the food textures they receive [32].

Early life experiences with a variety of textured foods is critical for both food acceptance and development of adequate oral feeding skills to process with more complex foods encountered in the adult diet [33]. Rejection of solid foods or a long-term preference for softer and smoother foods may also have an atrophic effect on the stomatognathic muscles and bones resulting in long-term poorer oral anatomy development and masticatory efficiency [34]. Studies in animals show that sustained consumption of a liquidised diet of puree foods can reduce masseter and temporalis muscle size and function, and impact motor development in the jaw and tongue [35]. In addition, chewing helps to increase mobility of the tongue and improve jaw coordination to ensure that complex textures can be moved between occlusal surfaces for crushing, and mastication approaches can be adapted to the changing textures experienced during food deformation. The timely introduction of developmentally appropriate textures can reduce the occurrence of feeding problems in later childhood such as aversions to textured foods (foods with 'bits' in them), and exclusive preferences for pureed food [36, 37]. Whereas younger children universally prefer smooth textures over lumpy textures with pieces, older children develop a preference for complex foods through repeated exposure to gradually lumpier foods and biphasic textures [19, 38]. Given the reciprocal relationship between the consumption of increasingly challenging textures and healthy oral development, it is important to avoid sustained consumption of softer diets and instead align developmentally appropriate textures with the child's developing oral anatomy, to enhance both feeding skills and texture acceptance in later childhood.

2.2.4 Eating Behaviours, Energy Intake and Growth During the Preschool Years (3–6 Years)

The emergence of dentition and feeding skills is followed by the development of food preferences and the stable eating behaviours that support daily food intake and dietary patterns associated with growth and body composition during early childhood [39]. In early life, differences emerge in eating behaviours that can track into later childhood and have a sustained impact on energy intake and weight gain [40]. These include differences in microstructural patterns of eating and specific eating behaviours such as eating rate, average bite size and chews per bite [41]. Early-life differences in eating behaviours have been associated with differences in growth and body composition in later childhood. For example, infants that display a higher nutritive suckling rate have been associated with increased weight gain in the first years of life [42, 43]. Children with obesity tend to eat more rapidly than non-obese children and exhibit these eating behaviours more consistently during the preschool years [44, 45]. One suggestion is that this could be a behavioural manifestation of an increased motivation or 'drive' to eat. The 'biobehavioural model' of obesity proposes that a child's risk of developing obesity is operational via a heightened appetitive response to their food environment [46, 47]. These appetite traits are captured by parent report using the child eating behaviour questionnaire (CEBQ) and reflect differences in children's underlying motivation to consume food. These differences in child appetitive traits are characterised by faster eating rates, poorer satiety responsiveness, and a higher food responsiveness and enjoyment of food [48].

The eating behaviours that stabilise in early life can track over time and may reflect a stronger appetite avidity, motivation to eat and decreased sensitivity to satiety signals during a meal, predisposing the child to higher energy intakes and increased risk of weight gain. Research on twins has shown a linear relationship between faster eating rates and higher weight gain, with an increase of 0.18 bites/min for each unit increase in body mass index among the children studied [49]. The same twin study has suggested that eating rate is a highly heritability behaviour and may be a phenotypic expression of an increased risk of excessive weight gain during childhood. In a prospective study, Berkowitz and colleagues showed that a faster eating style characterised by increased mouthful per minute was associated with greater prospective increases in BMI and adiposity [50]. Recent research from the Growing Up in Singapore Towards Healthier Outcomes (GUSTO) birth cohort in Singapore has shown a linear relationship between faster eating rates and energy intake (Fig. 2.1) with children that ate faster consuming up to 75% more energy within the same meal compared to children that ate at a slower rate [51]. Faster eating was also associated with higher child BMI scores, and increased adiposity at 4.5 years. The same children were again studied at 6 years of age where their faster eating rate at 4.5 years was a significant predictor of their eating rate and energy intake at the later time point. In addition, children that ate faster had higher increases in both BMI and adiposity compared to children that ate slower.

These findings highlight that once these eating behaviours become stable, they can have a sustained impact on energy intake and contribute to increased body weight and adiposity during childhood. This eating style has been described as 'obesogenic' and is characterised by larger average bite size, reduced chewing per bite and a shorter oro-sensory exposure time [41]. This obesogenic eating style supports increases in acute energy intake within a meal, and is more prevalent among, though not exclusive to, children with overweight and obesity. An obesogenic eating style is likely to continue into adulthood, where people who eat faster tend to consume more energy during a meal, and where longitudinal analysis of self-reported eating rate has been associated with increased risk of becoming overweight or obese, independently of other lifestyle factors [52]. In adults, eating rates have been shown to be highly consistent at an individual level and strongly predictive of energy intake from meal to meal [53]. This finding indicates that once an individual's habitual eating rate is

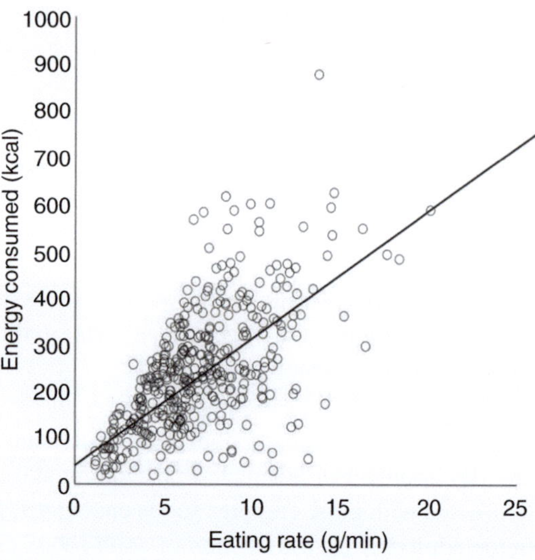

Fig. 2.1 Association between eating rate and energy intake during lunch ($r^2 = 0.38$, $p < 0.001$; n = 386) [51]

established, it is likely to remain consistent and 'automatic' over time, and can exert a sustained influence on their habitual energy intake [54].

The early-life influences that lead some children to consistently eat at a faster rate remain unclear, though it is likely a combination of both genetic predisposition and early-life environmental experience. Previous findings have suggested that eating rate is heritable and may be a phenotypic expression of an increased obesity risk. This may also be reflected in metabolic differences and research in adults has shown a positive relationship between higher basal metabolic rate and faster eating rates, suggesting that eating faster may be a behavioural adaptation to meet underlying increased energy demands [55]. Faster eating is likely to reflect a child's early-life experiences with foods, and may be linked with a heightened reactivity towards food stimuli. Research has shown that faster eating styles are more common among children with poorer trait inhibitory control, suggesting an association with higher executive functions linked with impulse control [56]. The early-life food environment and parental influences also play an important role in shaping young children's eating behaviours. During the preschool years, the family's diet, eating behaviours and parental feeding practices around mealtimes exert a significant influence on a child's experience with food, and the subsequent eating behaviours that emerge over time. Parents often use feeding practices around mealtimes to encourage, modify or restrict their child's food intake [57]. Research has shown that children that experience the most frequent feeding practices during meals tend to eat at a faster rate and consume significantly more energy than children who experience less frequent feeding practice. The use of feeding practices tended to be more frequent among girls than boys, although in both cases children that experience the most feeding practices consistently eat at a faster rate and consume more energy. Faster eating rates have been shown to mediate the relationship between appetitive traits linked with higher energy intakes, such that children with appetite traits associated with greater energy intakes typically only consume more energy when they also eat at a faster rate. Taken together these findings highlight the importance of early-life experiences with food and feeding practices during a period where the child's eating behaviours begin to stabilise, as once entrained, these behaviours are likely to remain consistent and contribute to habitual energy intakes over time.

Recognising children that display an obesogenic eating style is key to identifying those most at risk for obesity, and affords new opportunities to use eating behaviour strategies to mitigate the impact of faster eating on energy intake [40]. Longer oro-sensory exposure time can reduce the risk of overconsumption within a meal by promoting earlier termination of eating and by increasing inter-meal satiety [58]. Several interventions have attempted to retrain children's eating speed using devices that prompt or adjust eating rate during a meal. These approaches have yielded some success. In one example, children were shown to both reduce energy intake and reduce their BMI using a device that tracks eating speed against an eating rate target [59]. In a separate intervention, children were instructed to extend their inter-bite interval using a timer to slow eating rate and reduce energy intake. In a recent 8-week trial, children were provided with psycho-educational and behavioural techniques to slow their eating rate with results showing a reduction in eating speed and BMI and an increase in food enjoyment among children that successfully completed the intervention [57]. As highlighted earlier, children will adapt their oral processing behaviours to the textures of food served which creates the opportunity to reduce eating speed and energy intake by changing the texture of the child's diet. Research has compared the eating rate of different foods and found a 12-fold natural variation in the rate of consumption of solid foods and even larger variation in the consumption of semi-solid and liquid foods [60]. Texture-based differences in eating rate are due to the additional time required to mechanically deform a food structure, elasticity and stiffness and the need to adequately lubricate a food to form a swallowable bolus [61]. Experimental studies have manipulated food texture and shown that participants reduce their eating rate and decrease ad libitum energy intake by an average of 11–15%, potentially indicating a role for a food's sensory cues to support changes to eating behaviours [62–65]. A food-based approach to retraining children to eat at a slower rate has not yet been tested, but is appealing given the plasticity of food preferences at this age and the opportunity for the intervention to have an impact at every eating occasion.

These findings highlight the link between eating rate and obesity risk, and show that focusing on slowing eating rate may be an effective behavioural modification for family-based obesity prevention among children at high risk of developing obesity. Behavioural interventions have demonstrated some success although the long-term adherence and sustained impact of these programmes on habitual eating behaviour remain to be seen. Whereas identifying the maladaptive eating behaviours that sustain greater intakes provides improved diagnostic accuracy, it would be more effective to avoid their development entirely through the appropriate introduction of food textures and the transition to foods and eating behaviours that can support healthy growth and development.

2.3 Dietary Factors Affecting Nutritional Status in Children and Adolescents

The end result of the above oro-sensory development and learned eating behaviours is the consumption of combinations of foods or dietary patterns in childhood and adolescence. The food choices within such dietary patterns are essential to support growth and development but also directly influence nutritional status.

2.3.1 Dietary Patterns in Early Life and Adolescence

Adequate intake of all nutrients is essential to support growth and development. Initial dietary requirements are satisfied by bottle- or preferably breastfeeding but later supplemented with complementary foods as appropriate. Food-based dietary guidelines have been developed by most national competent authorities and by the World Health Organization to guide practical food choices and to ensure nutritional adequacy at all ages [66]. However, for many infants and young children, dietary intakes can deviate from that recommended. For example, in Europe inadequate dietary intakes can exist for nutrients such as alpha-linolenic acid, docosahexaenoic acid, iron, vitamin D and iodine, increasing the risk of inadequate status of these nutrients. Such shortfalls often exist alongside diets which are generally adequate for most nutrients except fibre and in some instances are relatively high in protein and salt [67]. During older childhood and in the teenage years, such suboptimal dietary patterns can continue and in Europe are characterised by excessive dietary intakes of saturated fat, free sugars and salt, and low fibre and lower intakes of nutrients such as iron, calcium, folate and vitamin A [68].

Specific mention is warranted for vitamin D, iron and folate. Low vitamin D status can affect all population groups whilst inadequate dietary iron and folate intakes are more likely in all young children and in teenage girls. For example, in the most recent waves of the United Kingdom National Diet and Nutrition Survey (NDNS), 10% of all 4–10-year-olds had circulating (blood)

levels of vitamin D suggestive of deficiency (<25 nmol/L), this figure rising to 26% of all 11–18-year-olds [69]. For iron, 54% of 11–15-year-old girls had dietary intakes below the reference amount that is only enough for a small number (2.5%) of people in the population (the Lowest Reference Nutrient Intake (LRNI)); that is, most people need more. Furthermore, low red blood cell folate status (indicative of anaemia; <305 nmol/L) was shown in 15–28% of all 11–18-year-old girls during the period 2014/2015 and 2015/2016 [69]. Inadequate folate intakes and status are of particular concern for teenage girls where adequate folate/folic acid intake is required to prevent neural tube defects where a pregnancy is unplanned. Such dietary patterns are reflected in many other countries and indicate dietary imbalances with potential longer term implications for general health.

2.3.2 Dietary Associated Practices Which Can Influence Food Choice and Intake Patterns in Childhood and Teenage Years

Dietary preferences and habits established early in life will influence eating behaviour in later life. As well as meeting immediate needs for growth and development, dietary intake in the formative years can influence future risk of chronic diseases including heart disease, type 2 diabetes, osteoporosis and some forms of cancer [70–73]. During the transition from childhood, through adolescence and into adulthood, individuals gradually assume autonomy over their food intake decisions. Diet quality often declines from childhood to adolescence with a notable rise in sugar intake and, particularly, increased consumption of sugar-sweetened beverages [74]. Children and adolescents are vulnerable to a number of immediate health problems as a result of not eating an energy-balanced, nutrient-rich diet. These health problems include micronutrient inadequacies or outright deficiencies such as iron-deficiency anaemia or rickets; for example, a study of hospital admissions for rickets in England in children younger than 15 years, from 1968 to 2011, noted an increase in hospitalisation rates for rickets in the 2000s [75]. The emergence of obesity in children, most commonly reflecting an over-reliance on energy-dense, high-fat, high-sugar foods, compounded inadequate physical activity.

Parents who follow a vegetarian or vegan diet may also provide the same for their children. Whilst these dietary patterns can be nutritionally complete, careful planning is required. In particular, children following a vegan diet may be vulnerable to low intakes of several micronutrients including calcium, iron, iodine and vitamin D and may be at increased risk of fractures if nutrients from meat, milk and dairy foods are not adequately provided [76]. As a rule, any diet that recommends excluding specific food groups or categories of foods will place an individual at greater risk of poor nutritional status unless the diet is carefully planned to ensure nutrient adequacy. This planning requires a relatively high level of health literacy and motivation.

Another source of nutritional vulnerability in children is picky eating which is particularly prevalent in children under 2 years old [77]. In terms of food intake, picky eating is usually characterised by low dietary variety and an unwillingness to eat a variety of foods and, as a result, low intakes of iron and zinc (associated with low intakes of meat, and fruits and vegetables) are of particular concern. To avoid long-term problems with eating and health, parents will benefit from support and advice to implement strategies that can ameliorate picky eating such as repeated exposures to unfamiliar foods, parental modelling of eating fruits and vegetables and unfamiliar foods, and creation of positive social experiences around mealtimes [78].

2.4 Other Conditions and Considerations That Can Influence Dietary Intakes and Nutritional Status During Childhood and Teenage Years

A number of other diet-related conditions may influence dietary intakes and health during childhood and teenage years including presence of food allergies, coeliac disease and eating disorders. The prevalence of food allergies in Europe is estimated to be 5.9% for self-reported food allergy and 0.9% for positive food challenge diagnosis [79]. Food allergies stimulate an immune response which can be life threatening and the only treatment is avoidance of the allergen; milk, egg, peanut, tree nuts, wheat, soy, fish and shellfish are responsible for most IgE-mediated allergic reactions. Avoidance diets can place children at risk of inadequate nutrient intake which, in turn, can affect growth [80]. An international survey of 430 patients from 12 allergy centres throughout the world reported that 9% had stunted growth, 6% were underweight and 3–5% were overweight [81]. In particular, cow's milk allergy is associated with growth impairment in children that persists through adulthood [52, 82]. The risks of nutrient inadequacy increase in children with two or more allergies and expert dietetic input is required to support the families of children who are diagnosed with food allergies [83].

In contrast, coeliac disease is an autoimmune disorder triggered by the ingestion of gluten, a protein found in wheat, rye and barley. Coeliac disease can be diagnosed at any age and ingestion of gluten damages the villi in the small intestine resulting in malabsorption of nutrients including iron, folic acid, calcium and fat-soluble vitamins. Treatment for coeliac disease is lifelong adherence to a gluten-free diet [84]. A gluten-free diet is achieved by consuming naturally gluten-free foods such as fruits, vegetables, meat, fish and eggs, along with the use of gluten-free substitutes for cereal-based foods such as gluten-free bread and pasta. In addition to clinically diagnosed coeliac disease, there has been an increase in the perception of gluten intolerance in the general population and, as a result, an increase in the number of people following a gluten-free diet and seeking gluten-free substitutes [85]. As indicated previously, excluding a food group or specific types of food from the diet places an individual at increased risk of nutritional inadequacy. An increasing range of gluten-free substitutes have become available in recent years; however, these products are often expensive and are not necessarily the same as their gluten-containing equivalents:

it has been noted that gluten-free substitutes can be higher in fat, sugar and salt and lower in protein and micronutrients [85]. Dietary vigilance is required to ensure that all traces of gluten are eliminated from the diet whilst ensuring that appropriate gluten-free foods are consumed to meet the requirements for macro- and micronutrients. This is particularly relevant for children and adolescents to ensure that growth and development are not adversely affected.

Finally, eating disorders can commonly manifest in late childhood and early adolescence with binge-eating disorder, bulimia nervosa and anorexia nervosa being the most common types [86]. Eating disorders are commonly associated with under- or over-nutrition. Anorexia nervosa can result in severe malnutrition and so can have a significant negative impact on oral health. Individuals who have bulimia nervosa are at increased risk of dental erosion owing to repeated exposure of the dentition to acidic gastrointestinal contents through episodes of regurgitation/purging. In all instances, input from a multidisciplinary team (including dietitians) is required to ensure adequate growth and development and return to health [87].

2.5 Conclusion

This chapter has described the stages of oral anatomy development and eating behaviours from early life to adolescence. It has discussed key dietary considerations which may affect oral health during these life stages which are underpinned by these essential requirements: (1) supporting healthy development which enables the infant to transition to a balanced diet and (2) need to focus on developing healthy eating patterns rich in nutrient-dense foods with appropriate energy, vitamins and minerals to support age-appropriate growth.

References

1. Monteiro POA, Victora CG. Rapid growth in infancy and childhood and obesity in later life - a systematic review. Obes Rev. 2005;6(2):143–54. https://doi. org/10.1111/j.1467-789X.2005.00183.x.
2. Druet C, Stettler N, Sharp S, et al. Prediction of childhood obesity by infancy weight gain: an individual-level meta-analysis. Paediatr Perinat Epidemiol. 2012;26(1):19–2. https://doi. org/10.1111/j.1365-3016.2011.01213.x.
3. Koletzko B, Godfrey KM, Poston L, et al. Nutrition during pregnancy, lactation and early childhood and its implications for maternal and long-term child health: the early nutrition project recommendations. Ann Nutr Metab. 2019;74(2):93–106. https://doi. org/10.1159/000496471.
4. Nicklaus S, Demonteil L, Tournier C. 8 - Modifying the texture of foods for infants and young children. In: Modifying food texture: sensory analysis, consumer requirements and preferences, vol. 2. Amsterdam: Elsevier; 2015. https://doi.org/10.1016/ B978-1-78242-334-8.00008-0.
5. Le Révérend BJD, Edelson LR, Loret C. Anatomical, functional, physiological and behavioural aspects of the development of mastication in early childhood. Br J Nutr. 2014;111(3):403–14. https://doi.org/10.1017/ S0007114513002699.
6. Loret C, Walter M, Pineau N, Peyron MA, Hartmann C, Martin N. Physical and related sensory properties of a swallowable bolus. Physiol Behav. 2011;104(5):855–64. https://doi.org/10.1016/j.physbeh.2011.05.014.
7. Harshaw C. Alimentary epigenetics: a developmental psychobiological systems view of the perception of hunger, thirst and satiety. Dev Rev. 2008;28(4):541–69. https://doi.org/10.1016/j.dr.2008.08.001.
8. Carruth BR, Ziegler PJ, Gordon A, Hendricks K. Developmental milestones and self-feeding behaviors in infants and toddlers. J Am Diet Assoc. 2004;104:s51–6. https://doi.org/10.1016/j.jada.2003.10.019.
9. van den Engel-Hoek L, van Hulst KCM, van Gerven MHJC, van Haaften L, de Groot SAF. Development of oral motor behavior related to the skill assisted spoon feeding. Infant Behav Dev. 2014;37(2):187–91. https://doi.org/10.1016/j.infbeh.2014.01.008.
10. Wee MSM, Goh AT, Stieger M, Forde CG. Correlation of instrumental texture properties from textural profile analysis (TPA) with eating behaviours and macronutrient composition for a wide range of solid foods. Food Funct. 2018;9(10):5301–12. https://doi. org/10.1039/c8fo00791h.
11. Stokes JR, Boehm MW, Baier SK. Oral processing, texture and mouthfeel: from rheology to tribology and beyond. Curr Opin Colloid Interface Sci. 2013;18(4):349–59. https://doi.org/10.1016/j. cocis.2013.04.010.
12. Green JR, Moore CA, Ruark JL, Rodda PR, Morvée WT, VanWitzenburg MJ. Development of chewing in children from 12 to 48 months: longitudinal study of EMG patterns. J Neurophysiol. 1997;77(5):2704–16. https://doi.org/10.1152/jn.1997.77.5.2704.
13. Matsuo K, Palmer JB. Anatomy and physiology of feeding and swallowing: normal and abnormal. Phys Med Rehabil Clin N Am. 2008;19(4):691–707. https://doi.org/10.1016/j.pmr.2008.06.001.
14. Pires SC, ERJ G, Caramez Da Silva F. Influence of the duration of breastfeeding on quality of muscle function during mastication in preschoolers: a cohort

study. BMC Public Health. 2012;12(1):934. https://doi.org/10.1186/1471-2458-12-934.

15. Wilson EM, Green JR. The development of jaw motion for mastication. Early Hum Dev. 2009;85(5):303–11. https://doi.org/10.1016/j.earlhumdev.2008.12.003.

16. Barlow SM. Central pattern generation involved in oral and respiratory control for feeding in the term infant. Curr Opin Otolaryngol Head Neck Surg. 2009;17(3):187–93. https://doi.org/10.1097/MOO.0b013e32832b312a.

17. Stolovitz P, Gisel EG. Circumoral movements in response to three different food textures in children 6 months to 2 years of age. Dysphagia. 1991;6(1):17–25. https://doi.org/10.1007/BF02503459.

18. Gisel EG. Effect of food texture on the development of chewing of children between six months and two years of age. Dev Med Child Neurol. 1991;33(1):69–79. https://doi.org/10.1111/j.1469-8749.1991.tb14786.x.

19. Lundy B, Field T, Carraway K, et al. Food texture preferences in infants versus toddlers. Early Child Dev Care. 1998;146(1):69–85. https://doi.org/10.1080/0300443981460107.

20. Stevenson RD, Allaire JH. The development of normal feeding and swallowing. Pediatr Clin North Am. 1991;38(6):1439–53. https://doi.org/10.1016/S0031-3955(16)38229-3.

21. Gisel EG. Chewing cycles in 2- to 8-year-old normal children: a developmental profile. Am J Occup Ther Off Publ Am Occup Ther Assoc. 1988;42(1):40–6. https://doi.org/10.5014/ajot.42.1.40.

22. Castelo PM, Gavião MBD, Pereira LJ, Bonjardim LR. Maximal bite force, facial morphology and sucking habits in young children with functional posterior crossbite. J Appl Oral Sci. 2010;18(2):143–8. https://doi.org/10.1590/S1678-77572010000200008.

23. Castelo PM, Gavião MBD, Pereira LJ, Bonjardim LR. Masticatory muscle thickness, bite force, and occlusal contacts in young children with unilateral posterior crossbite. Eur J Orthod. 2007;29(2):149–56. https://doi.org/10.1093/ejo/cjl089.

24. Castelo PM, Pereira LJ, Bonjardim LR, Gavião MBD. Changes in bite force, masticatory muscle thickness, and facial morphology between primary and mixed dentition in preschool children with normal occlusion. Ann Anat. 2010;192(1):23–6. https://doi.org/10.1016/j.aanat.2009.10.002.

25. Carlsson GE. Bite force and chewing efficiency. Front Oral Physiol. 1974;1:265–92. https://doi.org/10.1159/000392726.

26. Demonteil L, Tournier C, Marduel A, Dusoulier M, Weenen H, Nicklaus S. Longitudinal study on acceptance of food textures between 6 and 18 months. Food Qual Prefer. 2019;71:54–65. https://doi.org/10.1016/j.foodqual.2018.05.010.

27. Coulthard H, Harris G, Emmett P. Delayed introduction of lumpy foods to children during the complementary feeding period affects child's food acceptance and feeding at 7 years of age. Matern Child Nutr. 2009;5(1):75–85. https://doi.org/10.1111/j.1740-8709.2008.00153.x.

28. Gavião MBD, Raymundo VG, Rentes AM. Masticatory performance and bite force in children with primary dentition. Braz Oral Res. 2007;21(2):146–52. https://doi.org/10.1590/s1806-83242007000200009.

29. Harris G, Mason S. Are there sensitive periods for food acceptance in infancy? Curr Nutr Rep. 2017;6(2):190–6. https://doi.org/10.1007/s13668-017-0203-0.

30. Northstone K, Emmett P, Nethersole F. The effect of age of introduction to lumpy solids on foods eaten and reported feeding difficulties at 6 and 15 months. J Hum Nutr Diet. 2001;14(1):43–54. https://doi.org/10.1046/j.1365-277X.2001.00264.x.

31. Mason SJ, Harris G, Blissett J. Tube feeding in infancy: Implications for the development of normal eating and drinking skills. Dysphagia. 2005;20(1):46–61. https://doi.org/10.1007/s00455-004-0025-2.

32. Schwartz JL, Niman CW, Gisel EG. Chewing cycles in 4- and 5-year-old normal children: an index of eating efficacy. Am J Occup Ther Off Publ Am Occup Ther Assoc. 1984;38(3):171–5. https://doi.org/10.5014/ajot.38.3.171.

33. Blossfeld I, Collins A, Kiely M, Delahunty C. Texture preferences of 12-month-old infants and the role of early experiences. Food Qual Prefer. 2007;18(2):396–404. https://doi.org/10.1016/j.foodqual.2006.03.022.

34. Araujo DS, Marquezin MCS, Barbosa TDS, Gavião MBD, Castelo PM. Evaluation of masticatory parameters in overweight and obese children. Eur J Orthod. 2016;38(4):393–7. https://doi.org/10.1093/ejo/cjv092.

35. Liu ZJ, Ikeda K, Harada S, Kasahara Y, Ito G. Functional properties of jaw and tongue muscles in rats fed a liquid diet after being weaned. J Dent Res. 1998;77(2):366–76. https://doi.org/10.1177/00220345980770020501.

36. Illingworth RS, Lister J. The critical or sensitive period, with special reference to certain feeding problems in infants and children. J Pediatr. 1964;65(6):839–48. https://doi.org/10.1016/s0022-3476(64)80006-8.

37. Werthmann J, Jansen A, Havermans R, Nederkoorn C, Kremers S, Roefs A. Bits and pieces: Food texture influences food acceptance in young children. Appetite. 2015;84:181–7. https://doi.org/10.1016/j.appet.2014.09.025.

38. Schwartz C, Vandenberghe-Descamps M, Sulmont-Rossé C, Tournier C, Feron G. Behavioral and physiological determinants of food choice and consumption at sensitive periods of the life span, a focus on infants and elderly. Innov Food Sci Emerg Technol. 2018;46:91–106. https://doi.org/10.1016/j.ifset.2017.09.008.

39. Birch LL, Fisher JO. Development of eating behaviors among children and adolescents. Pediatrics. 1998;101:539–49.

40. Forde CG, Fogel A, Mccrickerd K. Nurturing a healthy generation of children: research gaps and opportunities. Nestlé Nutrition Institute Workshop Series. Basel, Switzerland: Karger Publishers; 2019.

41. Fogel A, Goh AT, Fries LR, et al. A description of an 'obesogenic' eating style that promotes higher energy intake and is associated with greater adipos-

ity in 4.5-year-old children: Results from the GUSTO cohort. Physiol Behav. 2017;176:107–16. https://doi.org/10.1016/j.physbeh.2017.02.013.

42. Stunkard AJ, Berkowitz RI, Stallings VA, Schoeller DA. Energy intake, not energy output, is a determinant of body size in infants. Am J Clin Nutr. 1999;69(3):524–30. https://doi.org/10.1093/ajcn/69.3.524.

43. Agras WS, Kraemer HC, Berkowitz RI, Hammer LD. Influence of early feeding style on adiposity at 6 years of age. J Pediatr. 1990;116(5):805–9. https://doi.org/10.1016/S0022-3476(05)82677-0.

44. Drabman RS, Hammer D, Jarvie GJ. Eating styles of obese and nonobese black and white children in a naturalistic setting. Addict Behav. 1977;2(2-3):83–6. https://doi.org/10.1016/0306-4603(77)90023-5.

45. Drabman RS, Cordua GD, Hammer D, Jarvie GJ, Horton W. Developmental trends in eating rates of normal and overweight preschool children. Child Dev. 1979;50(1):211–6. https://doi.org/10.1111/j.1467-8624.1979.tb02996.x.

46. Carnell S, Wardle J. Measuring behavioural susceptibility to obesity: validation of the child eating behaviour questionnaire. Appetite. 2007;48(1):104–13. https://doi.org/10.1016/j.appet.2006.07.075.

47. Syrad H, Johnson L, Wardle J, Llewellyn CH. Appetitive traits and food intake patterns in early life. Am J Clin Nutr. 2016;103(1):231–5. https://doi.org/10.3945/ajcn.115.117382.

48. Fogel A, Fries LR, McCrickerd K, et al. Oral processing behaviours that promote children's energy intake are associated with parent-reported appetitive traits: Results from the GUSTO cohort. Appetite. 2018;126:8–15. https://doi.org/10.1016/j.appet.2018.03.011.

49. Llewellyn CH, Van Jaarsveld CHM, Boniface D, Carnell S, Wardle J. Eating rate is a heritable phenotype related to weight in children. Am J Clin Nutr. 2008;88(6):1560–6. https://doi.org/10.3945/ajcn.2008.26175.

50. Berkowitz RI, Moore RH, Faith MS, Stallings VA, Kral TVE, Stunkard AJ. Identification of an obese eating style in 4-year-old children born at high and low risk for obesity. Obesity. 2010;18(3):505–12. https://doi.org/10.1038/oby.2009.299.

51. Fogel A, Goh AT, Fries LR, et al. Faster eating rates are associated with higher energy intakes during an ad libitum meal, higher BMI and greater adiposity among 4·5-year-old children: Results from the Growing Up in Singapore Towards Healthy Outcomes (GUSTO) cohort. Br J Nutr. 2017;117(7):1042–51. https://doi.org/10.1017/S0007114517000848.

52. Robinson E, Almiron-Roig E, Rutters F, et al. A systematic review and meta-analysis examining the effect of eating rate on energy intake and hunger. Am J Clin Nutr. 2014;100(1):123–51. https://doi.org/10.3945/ajcn.113.081745.

53. McCrickerd K, Forde CG. Consistency of eating rate, oral processing behaviours and energy intake across meals. Nutrients. 2017;9(8):891. https://doi.org/10.3390/nu9080891.

54. Ioakimidis I, Zandian M, Eriksson-Marklund L, Bergh C, Grigoriadis A, Södersten P. Description of chewing and food intake over the course of a meal. Physiol Behav. 2011;104(5):761–9. https://doi.org/10.1016/j.physbeh.2011.07.021.

55. Henry CJ, Ponnalagu S, Bi X, Forde C. Does basal metabolic rate drive eating rate? Physiol Behav. 2018;189:74–7. https://doi.org/10.1016/j.physbeh.2018.03.013.

56. Fogel A, McCrickerd K, Goh AT, et al. Associations between inhibitory control, eating behaviours and adiposity in 6-year-old children. Int J Obes. 2019;43(7):1344–53. https://doi.org/10.1038/s41366-019-0343-y.

57. Faith MS, Scanlon KS, Birch LL, Francis LA, Sherry B. Parent-child feeding strategies and their relationships to child eating and weight status. Obes Res. 2004;12(11):1711–22. https://doi.org/10.1038/oby.2004.212.

58. Zhu Y, Hsu WH, Hollis JH. Increasing the number of masticatory cycles is associated with reduced appetite and altered postprandial plasma concentrations of gut hormones, insulin and glucose. Br J Nutr. 2013;110(2):384–90. https://doi.org/10.1017/S0007114512005053.

59. Ford AL, Bergh C, Södersten P, et al. Treatment of childhood obesity by retraining eating behaviour: Randomised controlled trial. BMJ. 2010;340:b5388. https://doi.org/10.1136/bmj.b5388.

60. Ferriday D, Bosworth ML, Godinot N, et al. Variation in the oral processing of everyday meals is associated with fullness and meal size: a potential nudge to reduce energy intake? Nutrients. 2016;8(5):315. https://doi.org/10.3390/nu8050315.

61. Aguayo-Mendoza MG, Ketel EC, van der Linden E, Forde CG, Piqueras-Fiszman B, Stieger M. Oral processing behavior of drinkable, spoonable and chewable foods is primarily determined by rheological and mechanical food properties. Food Qual Prefer. 2019;71:87–95. https://doi.org/10.1016/j.foodqual.2018.06.006.

62. Forde CG, Bolhuis D, Thaler T, De Graaf C, Martin N. Influence of meal texture on eating rate and food intake: Results from three ad-libitum trials. Appetite. 2013;71:474. https://doi.org/10.1016/j.appet.2013.06.023.

63. Forde CG, van Kuijk N, Thaler T, de Graaf C, Martin N. Texture and savoury taste influences on food intake in a realistic hot lunch time meal. Appetite. 2013;60(1):180–6. https://doi.org/10.1016/j.appet.2012.10.002.

64. McCrickerd K, Lim CMH, Leong C, Chia EM, Forde CG. Texture-based differences in eating rate reduce the impact of increased energy density and large portions on meal size in adults. J Nutr. 2017;147(6):1208–17. https://doi.org/10.3945/jn.116.244251.

65. Mccrickerd K, Forde CG. Sensory influences on food intake control: Moving beyond palatability. Obes Rev. 2016;17(1):18–29. https://doi.org/10.1111/obr.12340.

66. Preparation and use of food-based dietary guidelines. World Health Organization technical report series. 1998.

67. European Commission. Scientific opinion on nutrient requirements and dietary intakes of infants and young children in the European Union. EFSA J. 2013;11(10):3408. https://doi.org/10.2903/j.efsa.2013.3408.

68. Buttriss JL, Welch AA, Kearney JM, Lanham SA. Public health nutrition. 2nd ed. Hoboken, NJ: Wiley; 2017.

69. Roberts C, Steer T, Maplethorpe N, et al. National diet and nutrition survey: results from years 7 and 8 (combined) of the Rolling Programme (2014/2015-2015/2016). England, UK: Public Health England; 2018.

70. Chung ST, Onuzuruike AU, Magge SN. Cardiometabolic risk in obese children. Ann N Y Acad Sci. 2018;1411(1):166–83. https://doi.org/10.1111/nyas.13602.

71. Weaver CM, Gordon CM, Janz KF, et al. The National Osteoporosis Foundation's position statement on peak bone mass development and lifestyle factors: a systematic review and implementation recommendations. Osteoporos Int. 2016;27(4):1281–386. https://doi.org/10.1007/s00198-015-3440-3.

72. Weichselbaum E, Buttriss JL. Diet, nutrition and schoolchildren: an update. Nutr Bull. 2014;39(1):9–73. https://doi.org/10.1111/nbu.12071.

73. Clarke MA, Joshu CE. Early life exposures and adult cancer risk. Epidemiol Rev. 2017;39(1):11–27. https://doi.org/10.1093/epirev/mxx004.

74. Mazarello Paes V, Hesketh K, O'Malley C, et al. Determinants of sugar-sweetened beverage consumption in young children: a systematic review. Obes Rev. 2015;16(11):903–13. https://doi.org/10.1111/obr.12310.

75. Goldacre M, Hall N, Yeates DGR. Hospitalisation for children with rickets in England: a historical perspective. Lancet 2014;383(9917):597–8. https://doi.org/10.1016/S0140-6736(14)60211-7.

76. Appleby P, Roddam A, Allen N, Key T. Comparative fracture risk in vegetarians and nonvegetarians in EPIC-Oxford. Eur J Clin Nutr. 2007;61(12):1400–6. https://doi.org/10.1038/sj.ejcn.1602659.

77. Cole NC, An R, Lee SY, Donovan SM. Correlates of picky eating and food neophobia in young children: A systematic review and meta-analysis. Nutr Rev. 2017;75(7):516–32. https://doi.org/10.1093/nutrit/nux024.

78. Taylor CM, Emmett PM. Picky eating in children: causes and consequences. In: Proceedings of the Nutrition Society; 2019. https://doi.org/10.1017/S0029665118002586.

79. Nwaru BI, Hickstein L, Panesar SS, et al. The epidemiology of food allergy in Europe: a systematic review and meta-analysis. Allergy Eur J Allergy Clin Immunol. 2014;69(1):62–75. https://doi.org/10.1111/all.12305.

80. D'Auria E, Abrahams M, Zuccotti G, Venter C. Personalized nutrition approach in food allergy: is it prime time yet? Nutrients. 2019;11(2):359. https://doi.org/10.3390/nu11020359.

81. Meyer R, Wright K, Vieira MC, et al. International survey on growth indices and impacting factors in children with food allergies. J Hum Nutr Diet. 2019;32(2):175–84. https://doi.org/10.1111/jhn.12610.

82. Sinai T, Goldberg MR, Nachshon L, et al. Reduced final height and inadequate nutritional intake in cow's milk-allergic young adults. J Allergy Clin Immunol Pract. 2019;7(2):509–15. https://doi.org/10.1016/j.jaip.2018.11.038.

83. Venter C, Mazzocchi A, Maslin K, Agostoni C. Impact of elimination diets on nutrition and growth in children with multiple food allergies. Curr Opin Allergy Clin Immunol. 2017;17(3):220–6. https://doi.org/10.1097/ACI.0000000000000358.

84. Lebwohl B, Sanders DS, Green PHR. Coeliac disease. Lancet. 2018;391(10115):70–81. https://doi.org/10.1016/S0140-6736(17)31796-8.

85. Pellegrini N, Agostoni C. Nutritional aspects of gluten-free products. J Sci Food Agric. 2015;95(12):2380–5. https://doi.org/10.1002/jsfa.7101.

86. Vo M, Accurso EC, Goldschmidt AB, Le Grange D. The impact of DSM-5 on eating disorder diagnoses. Int J Eat Disord. 2017;50(5):578–81. https://doi.org/10.1002/eat.22628.

87. Lo Russo L, Campisi G, Di Fede O, Di Liberto C, Panzarella V, Lo Muzio L. Oral manifestations of eating disorders: a critical review. Oral Dis. 2008;14(6):479–84. https://doi.org/10.1111/j.1601-0825.2007.01422.x.

Oral Health in Children

3

Joanna May

Abstract

Promoting good oral health in children encompasses preventing and controlling disease in a number of different structures including the oral mucosa, gingiva, periodontium and dental hard tissues. The most common cause of poor oral health in children is dental caries which can cause significant pain and discomfort. Caries development can be directly attributed to dietary factors and poor oral hygiene and can have a significant impact on the child's growth and development. Gingival and periodontal conditions are rarer in children and are usually related to either genetic or systemic conditions. The oral mucosa is directly related to the gastrointestinal mucosa as well as the skin and oral lesions can therefore help to diagnose systemic conditions such as infections, haematological oncology, anaemias, nutritional deficiencies and gastrointestinal conditions for example coeliac disease, ulcerative colitis and Crohn's disease.

J. May (✉)
Paediatric Dentistry, Alder Hey Children's Hospital,
Alder Hey Children's NHS Foundation Trust,
Liverpool, United Kingdom
e-mail: Joanna.may@nhs.net

3.1 Dental Caries

Dental caries is the episodic demineralisation and remineralisation of dental hard tissues by acid produced by plaque bacteria as a by-product of metabolism of dietary carbohydrates (Fig. 3.1). It is consistently found to be one of the most common preventable diseases worldwide with around 35% of the global population having untreated decay in the permanent dentition [1]. The caries process often starts in childhood with the National Health Service (NHS) Dental Epidemiology Programme in the United Kingdom reporting that 12% of 3-year-olds in England had experience of caries in the primary dentition in 2013. This increased to 23.3% of 5-year-olds surveyed in 2016/2017 and 34% of 12-year-olds had decay in their permanent teeth [2]. The prevalence of caries in under 6-year-olds is reported to be between 1 and 12% in higher income countries (3–6% in the United States, 11.4% in Sweden and 7–19% in Italy) but it is as high as 70% in lower income countries and amongst disadvantaged groups [3].

Evidence has shown that severe dental caries can contribute to failure to thrive in otherwise healthy children [4]. Untreated dental caries may affect children's nutrition causing pain when eating, food packing and difficulty chewing foods. Children's development can also be affected by poor sleep due to dental pain, chronic infection and missed education due to pain, sepsis and

G. McKenna (ed.), *Nutrition and Oral Health*, https://doi.org/10.1007/978-3-030-80526-5_3

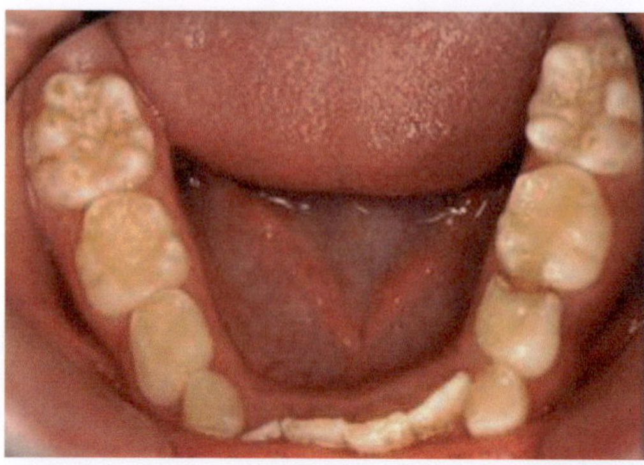

Fig. 3.1 Dental caries in lower deciduous teeth (clinical photo provided by Dr. Nora O'Murchu)

attendance at dental appointments. The United Kingdom Child Dental Health Survey 2013 reported that 22% of 12-year-olds and 19% of 15-year-olds reported difficulty eating in the past 3 months and 58% and 45% of 12- and 15-year-olds, respectively, reported that daily life had been affected by problems with their teeth and mouth [5, 6].

Several studies have shown a relationship between dental caries and educational attainment. Dental pain can lead to problems with concentration in school and to missed schooling. Children with poor oral health are nearly three times more likely to miss school due to dental pain and on average miss 1 day of school a year [7, 8]. They also report more problems at school, are less likely to complete homework and have lower self-esteem [8]. This translates into poorer outcomes, with children who had toothache in the last 6 months being 3.7 times more likely to have lower grades than those without toothache [9]. Once acute oral health problems are treated school performance and attendance improve [10]. Untreated dental caries can result in pulpal necrosis and development of a dental abscess in children. It is thought that chronic inflammation as a result of this form of dental infection may affect children's growth and development through the effect of cytokine release on erythropoiesis. For example, interleukin-1 inhibits erythropoiesis reducing erythrocyte production in bone marrow leading to less haemoglobin and chronic anaemia [11, 12]. Removal of this source of chronic inflammation may therefore increase haemoglobin levels and support the child's increased growth and development.

3.2 Sugar Intake and Caries

Dental caries is predominantly caused by frequent consumption of refined carbohydrates [13]. Dietary carbohydrate is a fundamental macronutrient and underpins food-based dietary guidelines globally. However, carbohydrate is a heterogeneous substance, composed of starches, sugars and various fibres. There is a significant body of evidence implicating sugars in the development of dental caries, particularly when frequently consumed [14–19]. In general terms, dietary sugars provide a food source for cariogenic bacteria normally present in the mouth, producing acid and lowering the pH in the oral cavity leaving the teeth vulnerable to decay. Frequent exposure leaves the teeth increasingly vulnerable. Table 3.1 summarises the various terms used to describe sugar as part of food-based dietary guidelines globally. Older definitions unique to the United Kingdom and which are now outdated are not described, e.g. non-milk extrinsic sugars. Whilst there is general consensus regarding use of the term 'total sugar', differences exist as to whether emphasis should be placed on the term 'free sugar' or 'added sugar'; the main difference between these two categories is that free sugar includes all naturally occurring sugars in non-intact (i.e. juiced or pureed) fruits and vegetables whereas 'added' sugar does not [23]. Unhelpfully, subtle differences also exist between the definitions of free sugar adopted by some authorities including the World Health Organization [20, 22]. Critically, for consumers (including parents and care providers for infants and young children), values stated on food labels reflect total sugar and typically do not differentiate between sugar types which may hinder understanding [23].

Early childhood caries (ECC) is defined as the presence of one or more decayed, missing or filled tooth surfaces in any primary tooth of children aged under 71 months [24]. Caries-related

Table 3.1 Summary overview of select definitions of sugar used in dietary guidance globally

Definition of sugar	World Health Organization [20]	United States [21]	European Union [19]	United Kingdom [14, 22]
Total sugar	Sum total of dietary sugars (mono- and disaccharides) present in food from any source	Sum total of dietary sugars (mono- and disaccharides) present in food from any source	Sum total of dietary sugars (mono- and disaccharides) present in food from any source	Sum total of dietary sugars (mono- and disaccharides) present in food from any source
Added sugar		Monosaccharides and disaccharides added during cooking or processing. It excludes naturally occurring sugars present in intact fruits, vegetables or dairy products or in juiced or pureed fruits and vegetables	Sucrose, fructose, glucose, starch hydrolysates (glucose syrup, high-fructose syrup) and other isolated sugar preparations used as such or added during food preparation and manufacturing. It excludes naturally occurring sugars present in intact fruits, vegetables or dairy products or in juiced or pureed fruits and vegetables	
Free sugar	Free sugars include monosaccharides and disaccharides added to foods and beverages by the manufacturer, cook or consumer. It excludes those naturally occurring and present in whole (intact, cooked or dried) fruits and vegetables or dairy products but includes sugars naturally present in honey, syrups, fruit juices and fruit juice concentrates			Free sugars include monosaccharides and disaccharides added to foods and beverages by the manufacturer, cook or consumer. It excludes those naturally occurring and present in whole (intact, cooked or dried) fruits and vegetables, cereal grains, seeds or dairy products but includes sugars naturally present in honey, syrups, fruit juices, fruit juice concentrates, purees, pastes or extrudates and lactose and galactose when added as an ingredient

dietary habits are established by 12 months of age and in very young children the main source of sugars within the diet comes from breast milk or drinks within feeding bottles [25]. A systematic review and meta-analysis of breast- and bottle feeding found that breastfeeding is more effective at preventing ECC than bottle feeding [26]. Alongside the other benefits of breastfeeding the World Health Organization therefore recommends exclusive breastfeeding up to 6 months of age, with continued breastfeeding together with appropriate complementary foods up to 2 years of age or beyond [27]. Breastfeeding for longer periods, over 12 months, reduces the risk of dental caries but breastfeeding overnight or ad libitum after 12 months of age increases the risk [26, 28]. In addition sleeping with a bottle, particularly one containing juice, has been found to be associated with high levels of dental caries in young children as does prolonged, frequent use of a bottle or sippy or non-spill cup [29]. Current recommendations are to encourage the use of a free-flow cup from 6 months of age and stop the bottle before the child's 1st birthday [30, 31].

Guidance from the World Health Organization advises limiting free sugar intake to less than 10% of total energy in all age groups, but ideally to less than 5% [20]. However it is well documented that dietary intakes of sugar by children and adolescents often exceed any sugar recommendation. Using the available data, a recent global review reported that the highest intakes of total sugars (up to 38% total energy) were by infants and young children <4 years reflecting intakes of lactose from milk but with intakes of added sugars highest in school-aged children and adolescents (up to 19% of total energy) compared to younger children or adults [17]. Where reported, adherence to the 5% free sugar recommendation was poor. For example, in Australia, 97% of children and teenagers aged between 4 and 18 years exceeded this recommendation with similar results reported elsewhere [32, 33]. Unfortunately, from a dental health perspective, frequency or periodicity of sugar consumption throughout the daily diet is less frequently described using such dietary data; that is, it is less clear whether the sugar is predominately consumed in bolus forms (e.g. at meals) or dispersed throughout the day (to include snacks). Analysis of contributing foods however does suggest that foods and drinks often consumed as snacks remain highly relevant including confectionery and sugar-sweetened beverages [16].

Frequent consumption of other dietary carbohydrates, particularly between meals, is also associated with dental caries in children. Dental caries and a poor diet are correlated with social deprivation but the easy availability of sugars and refined carbohydrates in foods and drinks in the Western diet has been linked with the current levels of dental decay in countries with less social deprivation. There has also been a rise in obesity in children in these countries. Although obesity and dental caries share many predisposing factors such as diet, lifestyle, genetics, socioeconomic status and other environmental factors, recent systematic reviews have found no definite association between body mass index (BMI) and dental caries [34]. However in the same meta-analysis there were higher levels of caries in primary and permanent teeth in the overweight and obese groups in high-income countries. Conversely,

malnutrition was also associated with ECC in preschool children and earlier studies found that children who required multiple extractions had lower body weight and failure to thrive [35, 36]. Differences in access to dental treatment between low- and high-income countries may therefore influence the impact of dental caries on weight. Studies in the Philippines, where 100% of 6-year-old children have dental caries, found that children had significantly greater weight gain after extraction of pulpally involved teeth under local anaesthetic and arresting caries in other teeth. There was no difference in height gain, therefore leading to an increased BMI [37].

3.3 Sugar Alternatives and Strategies to Reduce Intake

Given increased awareness and emerging science concerning the potential influence of sugar on health, there have been a number of initiatives to reduce dietary sugar intakes in children and younger adults, particularly those that deemed to be 'added' or 'free'. These could be broadly categorised as government or voluntary initiatives, with some overlapping activities. On a basic level, simple health promotion initiatives such as labelling or developing posters or physical models depicting the levels of sugar in foods and drinks commonly consumed by younger age groups can help educate both children and their parents/carers. The absence of sugar-containing options in vending machines or canteens along with the adoption of healthy eating policies is now more commonplace in preschools, schools, colleges and healthcare centres globally. More complex initiatives include taxation and food reformulation (either voluntary or mandatory) [33]. One consequence of reformulation is increased use of artificial sweeteners to impart sweetness and maintain food structure and texture at levels acceptable to consumers but without the associated calories. Both nutritive (bulk) and non-nutritive (intense) sweeteners are used by manufacturers, neither of which negatively impact on dental health. In the United States, the Food and Drug Administration has approved a 'does not promote tooth decay' health claim for sugar-free foods and beverages sweetened with the bulk sweetener sugar alcohol (e.g. polyols), with broadly similar claims relating to tooth mineralisation status approved for sugar alcohols in Europe [39]. However, given that initiatives to reformulate foods and reduce sugar intake are relatively recent, it is imperative that future surveys of both dietary sugar intake and dental health outcomes are completed to assess the impact and intakes of artificial sweeteners as well as sugars. Furthermore, irrespective of any such sugar reformulation, there is a continued need to focus on the development of healthy eating patterns in infants, young children and adolescents with the consumption of nutrient-dense foods filled with vitamins and minerals to support growth [40]. A summary of current best practice guidelines for diet and dental health from the United Kingdom is given in Table 3.2.

Table 3.2 Summary overview of best practice guidelines for diet and dental health from the United Kingdom [30, 38]

Dietary sugar
• To prevent dental decay, the amount and frequency of consumption of foods and drinks that contain free sugars should be reduced
• Sugar-free medicines should be recommended. If sugar-free is not available, take with meals if instructions allow and visit the dentist regularly
• Sugary food and drinks should only be consumed at mealtimes, if at all, rather than between meals. Mealtimes stimulate saliva production, which may help prevent tooth decay
Foods and drinks
• Because dried fruit can stick to the teeth it is better to consume it as part of a meal and not as a between-meal snack
• Choose fruits canned in juice rather than fruits in sugary syrup
• Fizzy drinks, soft drinks, juice drinks and squashes sweetened with sugar have no place in a child's daily diet
• Plain milk or tap water between meals is an ideal drink
Dental erosion
• Avoid frequent intake of acidic foods or drinks
• Keep acidic drinks to mealtimes and limit the number of fruit drinks (no more than one a day)
• Avoid acidic drinks at bedtime
• Fruit juice can cause dental erosion; only one glass (150 ml) of fruit juice can count as a portion of the five-a-day fruit and vegetable target
• Serve acidic drinks in a cup. They should not be sipped slowly or swished round the mouth as this increases contact time. If a straw is used, it should be placed behind the front teeth and well to the back of the mouth
• Drink acidic drinks ice cold
• Avoid brushing teeth for about an hour after consuming acidic drinks, since demineralisation of enamel occurs soon after drinking acidic drinks and makes the teeth more susceptible to abrasion
Dietary-associated practices
• Breastfeeding provides the best nutrition for babies
• From 6 months of age infants should be introduced to drinking from a free-flow cup, and from age 1 year feeding from a bottle should be discouraged
• Sugar should not be added to weaning foods or drinks. Encourage parents to make their own home-made weaning foods
• No solids or sugars should be added to a feeding bottle—bottles should only be used for expressed breast milk, infant formula or cooled boiled water
• Avoid sugar-containing foods and drinks at bedtime. During sleep salivary flow is low, and with swallowing decline this makes clearance of sugars in the mouth less frequent
• Infants should not be put to bed with a feeding bottle or feeder cup
• Babies/infants should have their teeth brushed before going to bed and not have any milk or anything else to drink or eat after brushing
• Soya-based infant formula should only be used under medical/dietetic/health visitor/public health nurse supervision
• Dummies or comforters should not be dipped into sugars, e.g. honey or sugary drinks
• A small cup of pure, unsweetened fruit juice can be given from the age of 6 months at mealtimes, diluted 50:50 with water, or with a greater proportion of water to juice if a longer more thirst-quenching drink is preferred
• To help prevent tooth decay, snacks should be nutritious and free from salt or free sugars

3.4   Dental Erosion

Whilst dental caries is described as the loss of tooth substance by acids formed by bacteria in dental plaque, dental erosion is described as the progressive irreversible loss of tooth substance by dietary acids. The estimated prevalence of erosive wear in the permanent teeth of children and adolescents is 30%, although there is high heterogeneity between studies [41]. Certain foods in the diet pose a risk for dental erosion owing to their acidic nature. Notably, dietary acids are found in fresh fruits and fruit juices, particularly citrus fruits and soft drinks. Carbonated soft drinks are a major contributor to dental erosion, even sugar-free varieties which are still acidic (Table 3.2). A case-control study of dietary factors associated with tooth erosion found that fruit intake between meals, but not with meals, was associated with erosive tooth wear, whereas acidic drinks maintained a strong association with tooth erosion regardless of whether they were consumed with or between meals [42]. A meta-analysis and meta-regression of the influence of diet in tooth erosion in children and adolescents found that carbonated drinks, acid sweets/sweets and natural acidic fruit juice were associated with an increase in erosion occurrence whilst milk and yoghurt reduced the likelihood of erosion occurrence [43]. Hence, advice is to limit fruit juice to one small glass a day and have it preferably with a meal as it also contains free sugars. Soft drinks should be avoided or only consumed as an occasional treat. NHS Health Scotland has noted in its oral health and nutrition guidance for health professionals: 'While it is recognised that excessive consumption of acidic fresh fruits, such as citrus fruit and apples, may cause dental erosion if eaten in large quantities, the individual and population health benefits of fruit consumption far outweigh any oral health detriments from these foods' [38].

3.5   Gingivitis and Periodontal Conditions

Poor plaque control is common in younger children and this is the most frequent reason for gingival inflammation. Children aged 8–14 years appear to accumulate plaque more rapidly and plaque control can be more difficult around exfoliating primary teeth and erupting permanent teeth with or without crowding. Increased gingival inflammation is also seen at puberty related to increased circulating sex hormones. Persistent gingivitis or bleeding gums despite improved oral hygiene or in the absence of dental infection or plaque can indicate serious systemic conditions including leukaemia and neutropenia. Children with red-purple, spongy, swollen gingiva and symptoms such as lethargy, malaise, sore throat, fever, skin infections that fail to heal, purpura, cervical lymphadenopathy, splenomegaly, hepatomegaly and petechiae should be referred for urgent blood tests and medical assessment.

Vitamin C deficiency (scurvy) can also cause inflammation and spontaneous bleeding of the gingival margins and papilla which have a bluish, soft, shiny, smooth appearance. This is a sign of severe undernutrition in children and is very rare in developed countries. However symptoms can be non-specific tiredness and weakness and the other connective tissue defects such as internal bleeding and impaired wound healing may be difficult to spot. Gingivitis, petechiae and a rash may therefore be the first indication of a deficiency.

Periodontal disease is rare in children and usually presents as aggressive periodontitis which can be localised (affecting incisors and first permanent molars) or generalised. There is often a genetic component to aggressive periodontitis and it is more common in African-Americans than White Europeans. It is characterised by early age of onset (before 30 years old), rapid periodontal destruction and low levels of plaque in relation to the extent of disease. Due to the rapid rate of destruction and risk of loss of permanent teeth at a young age, all children should have a periodontal screening carried out at dental examinations from the age of 7. A modified basic periodontal examination (BPE) should be undertaken until the permanent teeth are fully erupted at age 12 when a full BPE can be carried out [44].

Periodontal disease and early loss of teeth including primary teeth in children can be an indication of a localised lesion or systemic disease such as Papillon-Lefèvre, hypophosphatasia and leukocyte adhesion deficiency. Any child with these signs should be referred to a specialist as soon as possible for further investigation and management.

3.6 Soft-Tissue Lesions

Managing childrens' oral health also encompasses treatment for lesions of the soft tissues. The oral mucosa is an extension of the gastrointestinal tract internally and skin externally; thus conditions affecting either of these systems can also have effects on the oral mucosa. Often lesions in the oral cavity are the first sign of any systemic condition and can be invaluable in assisting with the diagnosis of gastrointestinal disorders as they can be seen without invasive techniques such as endoscopy and in a cooperative child a biopsy can be carried out under local anaesthetic eliminating the need for a general anaesthetic.

3.6.1 Recurrent Aphthous Ulceration

Recurrent aphthous ulcers (RAU) are relatively common in paediatric patients (34.9% in 15–16-year-olds) with onset typically occurring between 10 and 19 years old. RAU are defined as having a round, yellow-grey centre and erythematous halo [45]. They are classified as minor, major or herpetiform according to their size, healing and history. They should be distinguished from other forms of ulceration in children such as trauma, viral infections and those caused by multisystem, gastrointestinal or dermatological conditions such as Behcet's syndrome. There is often a genetic component to RAU in children with an increased prevalence and severity in children of parents with RAU as well as an earlier age of onset. Trauma and stress are also associated with increased RAU. This is particularly important for children and adolescents undertaking examinations. Studies have found an increase in frequency of ulcers during examination periods and a reduction during school holidays [46].

Deficiency of iron, folic acid and vitamin B12, all important in the production of haemoglobin and erythrocytes, has been linked with RAU. Children suffering with RAU should always be asked about their diet especially intake of foods high in iron, folic acid and vitamin B12 such as red meat, green vegetables, lentils and beans, cereals, citrus fruits, fish, poultry and eggs. Iron-deficiency anaemia may also be responsible for the onset of RAU in girls at the time of menstruation when their dietary intake of iron may be insufficient to replace menstrual blood loss. Field et al. found that 21% of 7–16-year-olds with RAU had some haematological anomalies, 5% had iron-deficiency anaemia and 13% had iron deficiency without anaemia. Seven of 100 children had anaemia suggestive of malabsorption and underwent jejunal biopsy but only one of these had findings consistent with a diagnosis of coeliac disease [47]. The recommendation is therefore to undertake haematological screening for children suffering with RAU as listed in Table 3.3. If there is a strong suspicion of malabsorption or coeliac disease then the serum immunoglobulin A (IgA) tissue transglutaminase (TTG) antibody test or the IgA-endomysial antibody (EMA) test as well as total serum IgA level should be undertaken before a biopsy. If coeliac disease is confirmed then the patient should be started on a gluten-free diet as soon as possible as adherence to this diet mostly leads to reduction or complete resolution of the oral ulceration [48].

Table 3.3 Recommended haematological screening for children with RAU

Haemoglobin concentration and red cell indices
Full blood count and differential white cell count
Erythrocyte sedimentation rate
Serum ferritin
Serum B12
Serum and red cell folate
If coeliac disease suspected: serum immunoglobulin A tissue transglutaminase (TTG) and total serum IgA

3.6.2 Oral Manifestations of Crohn's Disease

Crohn's disease is an inflammatory bowel disease with characteristic granulomatous inflammatory lesions occurring anywhere along the gastrointestinal tract from the mouth to anus. Oral signs of Crohn's disease include RAU, lip swelling, cobblestoning of the buccal mucosa, mucosal tags, linear ulcers and mucogingivitis. As discussed previously RAU and gingivitis can be indicative of a number of conditions but lip swelling, cobblestoning and mucosal tags should arouse a higher degree of suspicion of Crohn's disease.

Oral lesions are more common in younger patients; the average age at presentation is 12. The prevalence of oral lesions in diagnosed Crohn's disease varies between 0.5 and 48% with a higher prevalence of oral lesions found when oral examination was undertaken by paediatric dentists [49, 50]. Mucogingivitis was found in 17–60% of children with oral Crohn's, mucosal tags in 20–67%, labial swelling in 15–67%, cobblestoning in 8–15% and deep ulceration in 20% [33, 34]. When oral lesions in children were biopsied 75–100% had non-caseating granulomas which are diagnostic for Crohn's disease [49]. Patients are more likely to complain of oral symptoms than gastrointestinal symptoms and oral examination and biopsy are less invasive than endoscopies and gastrointestinal biopsies, particularly for children. Therefore anyone presenting with any gastrointestinal symptoms and possible diagnosis of inflammatory bowel disease should have an oral examination by a paediatric dentist and consider biopsy of any oral lesions found. This may enable a timely diagnosis of Crohn's disease and management of oral symptoms.

3.6.3 Recurrent Oral Infections

Oral infections, especially viral infections such as herpetic gingivostomatitis and hand, foot and mouth disease, are more common in young children than adults as their immune system is still developing. However recurrent, severe, unusual or prolonged oral infections including oral candidiasis may be an indication of an underlying immune deficiency. Primary immunodeficiencies including DiGeorge syndrome, severe combined immune deficiency and hyper IgE syndrome are inherited and present during first 2 years of life. Secondary immunodeficiencies occur well after infancy and include human immunodeficiency virus infection, malnutrition, malignancy, immunosuppressive medication, protein loss, asplenia, sickle cell disease, diabetes mellitus, severe liver disease and renal failure.

3.7 Defects of Dental Hard Tissues

Primary teeth begin to calcify between 3 and 6 months in utero with the crown completed between 1.5 months and 11 months old. Permanent teeth calcify from birth for first permanent molars to 2.5 years for second permanent molars with crowns completely formed by 3 years and 8 years, respectively. Therefore any systemic disruption such as hypoxia, infections, medication and nutritional deficiencies during these time periods can cause defects in the crown formation especially enamel hypoplasia. Defects in the enamel structure create an uneven surface and possibly sensitivity which leads to plaque retention and an increased risk of dental caries.

3.7.1 Vitamin D Deficiency

In cohort studies in the 1970s, Nikiforuk and Fraser found that children with disorders of calcium and phosphate metabolism, in particular hypocalcaemia, had increased levels of enamel hypoplasia [51]. They went on to determine that children with hereditary vitamin D-dependent rickets, hypoparathyroidism or pseudohypoparathyroidism had significant enamel hypoplasia in the permanent and sometimes primary dentition due to hypocalcaemia. In the same study children with hypophosphataemic rickets did not have enamel hypoplasia as although they have hypophosphataemia they have normal calcium levels [51].

Purvis, Mackay et al. also found that 56% of infants with neonatal tetany (caused by hypocalcaemia) later showed enamel hypoplasia of the primary dentition and this was related to the chronological period of tooth development in the 3 months prior to birth [52]. Maternal hypocalcaemia therefore has an effect on the occurrence of enamel hypoplasia in young children. Furthermore they found an inverse relationship between the mean hours of sunlight in the 3 months before birth and neonatal tetany suggesting that maternal vitamin D levels are important in the development of enamel defects. Schroth et al. found that 33% expectant mothers had deficient vitamin D and deficiency was more common in those with a due date in winter months. Twenty-two percent of their cohort of infants aged 1 year had evidence of enamel hypoplasia and 23% had cavitated ECC. They found significant relationships between ECC and enamel hypoplasia and maternal levels of vitamin D [53]. Vitamin D supplementation should be recommended for all pregnant women with increased risk of vitamin D deficiency, for example low sunlight hours, darker skin tones and vegetarian or vegan diets. Children who are exclusively breastfed after 6 months are also more susceptible to vitamin D deficiency especially those who are not exposed to much sunlight or have darker skin tones as their mothers are often unable to produce sufficient vitamin D to maintain both their own and their child's levels.

Interestingly Schroth et al. also found that optimal levels of vitamin D prenatally (>75 nmol/L) led to a reduced number of decayed teeth in the infants compared with lower levels of maternal vitamin D [53]. Systematic reviews have also found that vitamin D supplementation in children up to the age of 13 years led to a 47% reduced risk of dental caries suggesting that vitamin D may have a caries-preventive effect over and above the impact on enamel formation [54]. Vitamin D-dependent rickets is caused by impaired synthesis of 1,25-dihydroxy-vitamin D resulting in hypocalcaemia, elevated plasma parathyroid hormone concentration, hypophosphataemia and severe rickets despite sufficient intake of vitamin D. Hypocalcaemia usually occurs shortly after birth so second primary molars and permanent teeth can be affected by enamel hypoplasia. It can be effectively managed by supplementation with synthetic 1,25-dihydroxy-vitamin D.

Hypoparathyroidism is reduced or absent production of parathyroid hormone resulting in hypocalcaemia and hyperphosphataemia which can be either a permanent or a transient effect in the neonatal period. Pseudohypoparathyroidism is caused by a peripheral resistance to parathyroid hormone resulting in hypocalcaemia and hyperphosphataemia but normal or increased levels of parathyroid hormone. It usually presents later in life (mean age 5 years) so primary teeth and permanent incisors and first permanent molars are unlikely to be affected by hypoplasia. It can be treated with synthetic vitamin D and calcium supplements. Hypophosphataemic rickets is a genetic abnormality of renal tubular transport of phosphate leading to short stature, bow legs and abnormalities of enamel and pulp chambers which result in pulp exposure and spontaneous abscesses in the absence of dental caries. Primary teeth are often lost early.

Children diagnosed with any of these disorders should be advised of the possible effect on their dentition and advised to see a dentist from an early age (as soon as the first tooth erupts). Preventive dental advice should be given early, including twice-daily toothbrushing with a fluoride toothpaste and reduced frequency of sugar intakes to reduce the incidence of ECC. Similarly enamel hypoplasia in the primary dentition in the absence of these diagnoses should be investigated with a full prenatal and postnatal history and, if appropriate, blood tests including serum calcium, serum phosphorous, serum alkaline phosphatase and parathyroid hormone. This will enable early treatment with appropriate supplements or medications and prevent long-term effects on not only teeth but also skeletal growth and general health.

3.7.2 Coeliac Disease

Coeliac disease which develops before the age of 7 is associated with enamel hypoplasia in the permanent dentition as well as oral ulceration. The enamel hypoplasia tends to be symmetrical and chronological in all four quadrants and it most commonly affects incisors and molars. Often teeth have intact cusps with a band of hypoplasia just below the occlusal surface, reflecting the stage of development of the teeth when gastrointestinal symptoms presented and before gluten was eliminated from the diet. The prevalence of enamel defects in the permanent dentition ranges from 9.5% to 95.9% (mean 51.1%) and in primary teeth 5.8% to 13.3% (mean 9.6%) [40]. It is therefore more common than other oral mucosal lesions such as RAU in patients with coeliac disease. The effect on enamel may be due to gluten-induced immune-mediated damage to ameloblasts explaining the effect on the primary dentition or nutritional deficiencies particularly hypocalcaemia [55]. For this reason it is recommended that coeliac disease is considered as a possible diagnosis for any child presenting with this pattern of enamel hypoplasia. The child and parents should be asked about gastrointestinal symptoms such as pain, diarrhoea and weight loss as well as poor growth and fatigue. Any history of other autoimmune diseases such as diabetes and thyroiditis and family history of coeliac disease should also be investigated. If there is any suspicion of coeliac disease the child should be referred to a medical specialist for serum IgA-TTG antibody test [55].

3.8 Conclusion

Oral health in children has been viewed as an indicator of overall health, with poor oral health affecting a child's ability to learn, thrive, develop and potentially grow. The relationship between nutrition and oral health is interconnected as adequate nutrition is essential for optimal growth and oral health whilst poor oral health, specifically toothache and infection, can result in inadequate nutrition which may impact weight gain and growth. The mouth can also act as a reflection of the overall health of the child: soft-tissue lesions and dental enamel defects can provide vital information about the child's nutritional status or be the first signs of systemic illness. These lesions are easy to investigate without invasive procedures and can be key for early diagnosis and treatment of significant systemic conditions.

References

1. Marcenes W, Kassebaum NJ, Bernabé E, et al. Global burden of oral conditions in 1990-2010: a systematic analysis. J Dent Res. 2013;92(7):592–7. https://doi.org/10.1177/0022034513490168.
2. Public Health England. National Dental Epidemiology Programme for England: oral health survey of five-year-old children 2017 a report on the inequalities found in prevalence and severity of dental decay. England, UK: Public Health England; 2018.
3. Anil S, Anand PS. Early childhood caries: prevalence, risk factors, and prevention. Front Pediatr. 2017;2017:1415873. https://doi.org/10.3389/fped.2017.00157.
4. Elice CE, Fields HW. Failure to thrive: review of the literature, case reports, and implications for dental treatment. Pediatr Dent. 1990;12(3):185–9.
5. Tsakos G, Hill K, Chadwick B, Anderson T. Children's dental health survey 2013. Report 1: Attitudes, Behaviours and Children's dental health: England, Wales and Northern Ireland. Leeds, UK: Health and Social Care Information Centre; 2015.
6. Pitts N, Chadwick B, Anderson T. Child dental health survey 2013. Report 2: dental disease and damage in children. Leeds, UK: Health and Social Care Information Centre; 2015.
7. Jackson SL, Vann WF, Kotch JB, Pahel BT, Lee JY. Impact of poor oral health on children's school attendance and performance. Am J Public Health. 2011;101(10):1900–6. https://doi.org/10.2105/AJPH.2010.200915.
8. Guarnizo-Herreño CC, Wehby GL. Children's dental health, school performance, and psychosocial well-being. J Pediatr. 2012;161(6):1153–9. https://doi.org/10.1016/j.jpeds.2012.05.025.
9. Seirawan H, Faust S, Mulligan R. The impact of oral health on the academic performance of disadvantaged children. Am J Public Health. 2012;102(9):1729–34. https://doi.org/10.2105/AJPH.2011.300478.

10. White H, Lee JY, Vann WF. Parental evaluation of quality of life measures following pediatric dental treatment using general anesthesia. Anesth Prog. 2003;50:105–10.

11. Means RT, Krantz SB. Progress in understanding the pathogenesis of the anemia of chronic disease. Blood. 1992;80(7):1639–47. https://doi.org/10.1182/blood. v80.7.1639.bloodjournal8071639.

12. Means RT. Recent developments in the anemia of chronic disease. Curr Hematol Rep. 2003;2(2):116–21.

13. Moynihan P. Sugars and dental caries: Evidence for setting a recommended threshold for intake. Adv Nutr. 2016;7(1):149–56. https://doi.org/10.3945/ an.115.009365.

14. Scientific Advisory Committee on Nutrition. Carbohydrates and health. London: The Stationery Office; 2015.

15. Zhou SJ, Gibson RA, Gibson RS, Makrides M. Nutrient intakes and status of preschool children in Adelaide, South Australia. Med J Aust. 2012;196(11):696–700. https://doi.org/10.5694/ mja11.11080.

16. Buttriss JL, Welch AA, Kearney JM, Lanham SA. Public health nutrition. 2nd ed. Hoboken, NJ: Wiley; 2017.

17. Roberts C, Steer T, Maplethorpe N, et al. National diet and nutrition survey: results from years 7 and 8 (combined) of the rolling programme (2014/2015-2015/2016). England, UK: Public Health England; 2018.

18. Halvorsrud K, Lewney J, Craig D, Moynihan PJ. Effects of starch on oral health: systematic review to inform WHO guideline. J Dent Res. 2019;98(1):46–53. https://doi.org/10.1177/0022034518788283.

19. European Food Safety Authority. Scientific opinion on dietary reference values for carbohydrates and dietary fibre. EFSA J. 2010;8(3):1462.

20. World Health Organization. World Health Organization Guideline: Sugars intake for adults and children. World Health Organization Library Cat Data. 2015.

21. Nutrition Today. Agriculture USD of H and HS and USD of 2015 – 2020 Dietary Guidelines for Americans. In: 2015 – 2020 Dietary Guidelines for Americans. 8th ed; 2015. p. 18. https://doi. org/10.1097/NT.0b013e31826c50af.

22. Swan GE, Powell NA, Knowles BL, Bush MT, Levy LB. A definition of free sugars for the UK. Public Health Nutr. 2018;21(9):1636–8. https://doi. org/10.1017/S136898001800085X.

23. Mela DJ, MWoolner E. Perspective: total, added, or free? What kind of sugars should we be talking about? Adv Nutr. 2018;9(2):63–9. https://doi.org/10.1093/ advances/nmx020.

24. American Academy of Pediatric Dentistry. Policy on early childhood caries (ECC): classifications, consequences, and preventive strategies. Pediatr Dent. 2018;38(6):52–4.

25. Kranz S, Smiciklas-Wright H, Francis LA. Diet quality, added sugar, and dietary fiber intakes in American preschoolers. Pediatr Dent. 2006;28(2):164–71.

26. Avila WM, Pordeus IA, Paiva SM, Martins CC. Breast and bottle feeding as risk factors for dental caries: a systematic review and meta-analysis. PLoS One. 2015;10(11):e0142922. https://doi.org/10.1371/journal.pone.0142922.

27. World Health Organisation. Global strategy for infant and young child feeding. Geneva, Switzerland: World Health Organisation; 2003.

28. Reisine S, Douglass JM. Psychosocial and behavioral issues in early childhood caries. Commun Dent Oral Epidemiol. 1998;26:32–44. https://doi. org/10.1111/j.1600-0528.1998.tb02092.x.

29. Tinanoff N, Kanellis MJ, Vargas CM. Current understanding of the epidemiology, mechanisms, and prevention of dental caries in preschool children. Pediatr Dent. 2002;24(6):543–51.

30. Public Health England. Delivering better oral health: an evidence-based toolkit for prevention Summary guidance tables. London: Public Health England; 2014.

31. American Academy of Pediatric Dentistry. Policy on oral health care programs for infants, children, and adolescents. Pediatr Dent. 2018;30:21.

32. Australian Bureau of Statistics. Australian Health Survey: Consumption of food groups from the Australian dietary guidelines. Cat No 4364055012. 2016.

33. Public Health England. Sugar Reduction: Report on Progress between 2015 and 2018 September 2019; 2020.

34. Chen D, Zhi Q, Zhou Y, Tao Y, Wu L, Lin H. Association between dental caries and BMI in children: a systematic review and meta-analysis. Caries Res. 2018;52(3):230–45. https://doi. org/10.1159/000484988.

35. Janakiram C, Antony B, Joseph J. Association of undernutrition and early childhood dental caries. Indian Pediatr. 2018;55(8):683–5. https://doi. org/10.1007/s13312-018-1359-4.

36. Ayhan H, Suskan E, Yildirim S. The effect of nursing or rampant caries on height, body weight and head circumference. J Clin Pediatr Dent. 1996;20(3):209–12.

37. Monse B, Duijster D, Sheiham A, Grijalva-Eternod CS, Van Palenstein HW, Hobdell MH. The effects of extraction of pulpally involved primary teeth on weight, height and BMI in underweight Filipino children. A cluster randomized clinical trial. BMC Public Health. 2012;12:725. https://doi. org/10.1186/1471-2458-12-725.

38. National Health Service. Oral Health and Nutrition Guidance for Professionals Quick Reference Guide. Heal Scotland. 2012.

39. European Food Safety Authority (EFSA). Scientific Opinion on the substantiation of health claims related to the sugar replacers xylitol, sorbitol, mannitol, maltitol, lactitol, isomalt, erythritol, D-tagatose, isomaltulose, sucralose and polydextrose and maintenance of tooth mineralisation by decreasing tooth demineralisation. EFSA J. 2011;9(4):2076. https:// doi.org/10.2903/j.efsa.2011.2076.

40. Touger-Decker R, Mobley C. Position of the academy of nutrition and dietetics: oral health and nutrition.

J Acad Nutr Diet. 2013;113(5):693–701. https://doi.org/10.1016/j.jand.2013.03.001.

41. Salas MMS, Nascimento GG, Huysmans MC, Demarco FF. Estimated prevalence of erosive tooth wear in permanent teeth of children and adolescents: an epidemiological systematic review and meta-regression analysis. J Dent. 2015;43(1):42–50. https://doi.org/10.1016/j.jdent.2014.10.012.

42. O'Toole S, Bernabé E, Moazzez R, Bartlett D. Timing of dietary acid intake and erosive tooth wear: a case-control study. J Dent. 2017;56:99–104. https://doi.org/10.1016/j.jdent.2016.11.005.

43. Salas MMS, Nascimento GG, Vargas-Ferreira F, Tarquinio SBC, Huysmans MCDNJM, Demarco FF. Diet influenced tooth erosion prevalence in children and adolescents: results of a meta-analysis and meta-regression. J Dent. 2015;43(8):865–75. https://doi.org/10.1016/j.jdent.2015.05.012.

44. Clerehugh V, Kindelan S. Guidelines for periodontal screening and management of children and adolescents under 18 years of age. Br Soc Periodontol Br Soc Paediatr Dent. 2012;1–25. http://www.bsperio.org.uk/publications/downloads/54_090016_bsp_bspd-perio-guidelines-for-the-under-18s-2012.pdf.

45. Field EA, Brookes V, Tyldesley WR. Recurrent aphthous ulceration in children—a review. Int J Paediatr Dent. 1992;2(1):1–10. https://doi.org/10.1111/j.1365-263X.1992.tb00001.x.

46. Ship II, Morris AW, Durocher RT, Burket LW. Recurrent aphthous ulcerations and recurrent herpes labialis in a professional school student population. II. Medical history. Oral Surg Oral Med Oral Pathol. 1960;13(11):1317–29. https://doi.org/10.1016/0030-4220(60)90294-2.

47. Field EA, Rotter E, Speechley JA, Tyldesley WR. Clinical and haematological assessment of children with recurrent aphthous ulceration. Br Dent J. 1987;163(1):19–22. https://doi.org/10.1038/sj.bdj.4806174.

48. Campisi G, Di Liberto C, Carroccio A, et al. Coeliac disease: oral ulcer prevalence, assessment of risk and association with gluten-free diet in children. Dig Liver Dis. 2008;40(2):104–7. https://doi.org/10.1016/j.dld.2007.10.009.

49. Harty S, Fleming P, Rowland M, et al. A prospective study of the oral manifestations of Crohn's disease. Clin Gastroenterol Hepatol. 2005;3(9):886–91. https://doi.org/10.1016/S1542-3565(05)00424-6.

50. Pittock S, Drumm B, Fleming P, et al. The oral cavity in Crohn's disease. J Pediatr. 2001;138(5):767–71. https://doi.org/10.1067/mpd.2001.113008.

51. Nikiforuk G, Fraser D. The etiology of enamel hypoplasia: a unifying concept. J Pediatr. 1981;98(6):888–93. https://doi.org/10.1016/S0022-3476(81)80580-X.

52. Purvis RJ, Mackay GS, Cockburn F, et al. Enamel hypoplasia of the teeth associated with neonatal tetany: a manifestation of maternal vitamin-D deficiency. Lancet. 1973;2(7833):811–4. https://doi.org/10.1016/S0140-6736(73)90857-X.

53. Schroth RJ, Lavelle C, Tate R, Bruce S, Billings RJ, Moffatt MEK. Prenatal vitamin D and dental caries in infants. Pediatrics. 2014;133(5):e1277–84. https://doi.org/10.1542/peds.2013-2215.

54. Hujoel PP. Vitamin D and dental caries in controlled clinical trials: systematic review and meta-analysis. Nutr Rev. 2013;71(2):88–97. https://doi.org/10.1111/j.1753-4887.2012.00544.x.

55. Pastore L, Carroccio A, Compilato D, Panzarella V, Serpico R, Muzio L. Oral manifestations of celiac disease. J Clin Gastroenterol. 2008;42(3):224–32. https://doi.org/10.1097/MCG.0b013e318074dd98.

The Oral Health of the Ageing Population

4

Gerry McKenna, Murali Srinivasan, Claudio Leles, and Martin Schimmel

Abstract

Worldwide, the population is ageing. In many higher income countries, as birth rates fall and life expectancy increases, the proportion of older adults within the general population has increased. This has been one of the most distinctive demographic events of the last century and is predicted to continue at pace in the twenty-first century. Alongside population ageing, the oral health of older adults has also changed markedly with the emergence of a partially dentate older population. As patients retain more of their natural teeth for longer this does present challenges for the dental profession. Whilst construction of complete replacement dentures previously dominated oral care for older adults, prevention and management of chronic dental diseases are now increasingly important. Unfortunately this means that the burden of oral healthcare for the ageing population is also rising sharply and as oral health conditions exert an excessive burden on older adults, oral health inequalities have become a major concern. In this chapter, we discuss the impact of changing population and oral epidemiology on oral healthcare provision for older adults.

G. McKenna (✉)
Centre for Public Health, School of Medicine, Dentistry and Biomedical Sciences, Queen's University Belfast, Belfast, United Kingdom
e-mail: g.mckenna@qub.ac.uk

M. Srinivasan
Clinic of General, Special Care and Geriatric Dentistry, Centre of Dental Medicine, University of Zurich, Zurich, Switzerland

C. Leles
Department of Prevention and Oral Rehabilitation, School of Dentistry, Federal University of Goias, Goiânia, Brazil

M. Schimmel
Department of Reconstructive Dentistry and Gerodontology, School of Dental Medicine, University of Bern, Bern, Switzerland

4.1 General Population Demographics

Fertility rates have fallen in many higher income countries to below replacement levels as modern social changes impact behaviours. To date, fertility decline has been the main determinant of population ageing especially in higher income countries with the global fertility rate halving over the last 50 years. In future the transition towards lower fertility levels is expected to continue in the lower income countries, and to increase slightly in higher income countries. As fertility rates move towards lower levels, increased life expectancies assume an increasingly important role in population ageing. In higher income countries, where low fertility has

G. McKenna (ed.), *Nutrition and Oral Health*, https://doi.org/10.1007/978-3-030-80526-5_4

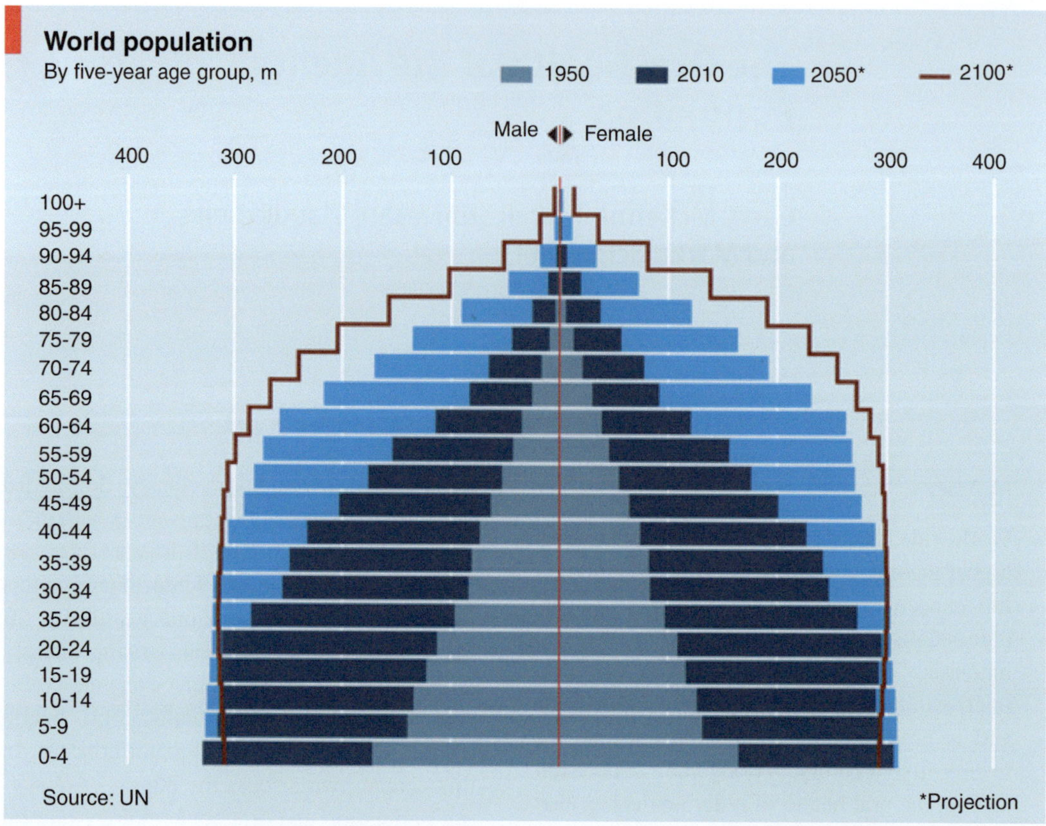

Fig. 4.1 Population demographic trends 1950–2100 [2]

prevailed for a significant period of time, relative increases in the older population are now principally determined by improved chances of surviving into old age [1]. Over the last five decades, life expectancy at birth has increased globally by almost 20 years. On average, the gain in life expectancy at birth was 23.1 years in lower income regions and 9.4 years in higher income regions. Over the next 50 years, life expectancy at birth is projected to increase globally by 10 years, to reach 76 years in 2050 (Fig. 4.1). As mortality becomes more concentrated at older ages of the population, the gap in life expectancy among regions is projected to decrease. By the end of the next quarter century, life expectancy at birth is expected to reach on average 80 years in the higher income regions and 71 years in lower income regions. In 2010, there were an estimated 524 million people aged over 65 years worldwide, and this number is expected to triple to

approximately 1.5 billion by 2050, accounting for nearly one-sixth of the global population [2]. These changes are occurring across the globe, as shown in Fig. 4.2, although the reasons for the changing population structure can differ, depending on the stage of demographic and epidemiologic transition.

4.2 Consequences of Changing Population Demographics

As a result of the generalised shift in the age distribution of mortality towards older groups, more people in future will survive into their seventh, eighth and ninth decades. Under current mortality conditions, almost three of every four newborns worldwide will survive to 60 years and approximately one of every three will live to over 80 years. Not only are more people surviving to

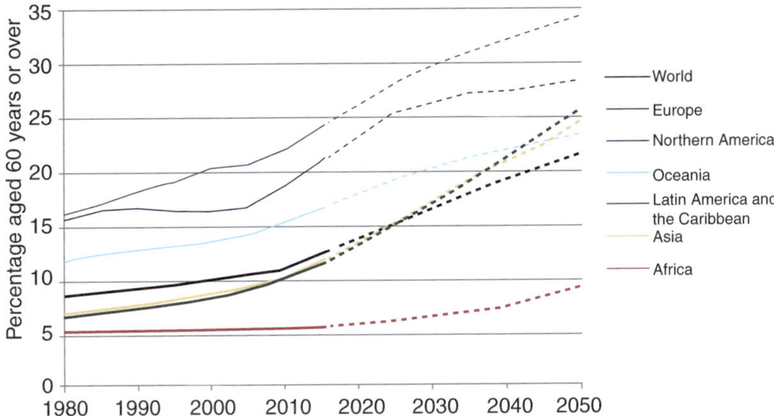

Fig. 4.2 Percentage of the global population aged 60 years and older [2]

old age, but once there, they tend to live longer. In the higher income regions, average life expectancy at age 80 is projected to increase by 27% over the next half century as compared with 19% at age 60 and 9% at birth [2]. The reasons for these improvements in life expectancy vary between countries but generally include increasing prosperity, education, public hygiene, improvements to housing and social welfare policies. However, progression in healthcare provision and treatment has also played an important role. Advances in preventative medicine, pharmaceuticals, imaging and medical technology have all contributed but have come with significant economic costs [3]. The result is that many older patients avail of increasingly expensive medical interventions and drugs. This has significant implications for government-funded healthcare as typically older patients no longer contribute to the tax base but are instead economically dependent on the state. In the United Kingdom, the Royal Commission on Long Term Care has estimated that the costs of caring for older adults will more than quadruple in real terms between 1995 and 2051, from £11.1 billion to £45.3 billion [4].

4.3 Systemic Comorbidity

An ageing population impacts society not only at a socio-economic level, but also from a biological viewpoint. Age-related changes effect functional and structural changes on the body, affecting all organ systems [5]. Functionality of organ systems declines and degenerative changes are evident in the skin and the musculoskeletal system [6]. These changes can markedly impact areas including general mobility and metabolism. For many older patients treatment rationale therefore shifts towards a preventive and/or a less invasive approach with the focus aimed at delaying or reversing some age-related changes on the body.

Amongst older patients, the prevalence of chronic medical conditions is very high with significant levels of comorbidity reported [7, 8]. Chronic diseases are conditions of long duration and generally slow progression which means that older adults are prone to compromised health, and often present with multi-morbid health status. Multi-morbidity is the presence of two or more chronic diseases requiring medication [9]. Common chronic diseases include heart disease, stroke, cancer, respiratory diseases and diabetes. They are the leading cause of mortality worldwide and currently account for 63% of all deaths [10]. By their nature, chronic diseases are significantly more prevalent amongst older patients. Of the 36 million people who died worldwide from chronic disease in 2008, only nine million were aged 60 years or less [11]. Management of multi-morbidity necessitates treatment which can impact oral health and the condition of the mouth and associated structures.

Xerostomia (dry mouth) is a common side effect of many drugs taken by older patients to control systemic medical conditions. In cases where patients require treatment to manage multiple chronic systemic diseases they are often prescribed multiple medications. Given the huge spectrum of drugs which cause hyposalivation, including tricyclic antidepressants, beta blockers and antihistamines, dry mouth is a common complaint in this patient group. A lack of saliva can have a devastating effect on the remaining dentition, directly contributing to an increased risk of caries, periodontal disease and subsequent tooth loss [12–14]. Xerostomia can also cause significant discomfort, make denture wearing very difficult and negatively impacting on quality of life [15].

Loss of autonomy with/without functional and cognitive decline may also be present in older adults. Dementia is common in older adults, especially in care-dependent patients within residential care [16]. An estimated 35.6 million people live with dementia worldwide, with the numbers expected to double every 20 years. Cognitive decline is considered one of the biggest health hazards in older adults, with a 50% incidence of Alzheimer's disease in those aged 85 years and over [16].

4.4 Oral Epidemiology

Consistent findings from epidemiological dental surveys indicate that tooth retention has increased in older patients as they retain more natural teeth into old age (Fig. 4.3) [17, 18]. Unfortunately, the cumulative nature of the two main destructive dental diseases, caries and periodontal disease,

dictates that ageing is always likely to be a factor associated with total tooth loss.

4.4.1 Trends in Edentulism

Although the overall prevalence of total tooth loss has fallen sharply over recent decades, patients are now becoming edentulous at an older age when they are generally less able to adapt to the limitations of complete dentures. The attitudes of older patients to oral health also appear to have changed as many take advantage of widely available sources of information and demand more conservative approaches to care from the dental profession, including retention of natural teeth. As a result, fewer patients are accepting of treatment simply centred around extractions and subsequent replacement of natural teeth [19].

A number of epidemiological surveys have demonstrated a strong socio-economic gradient amongst the population where the proportion of edentulous adults was considerably higher amongst lower socio-economic groups [20]. These findings have been demonstrated in the United Kingdom, Ireland, Japan and South Korea which found that socio-economic class has a profound effect on oral health behaviours and status [21]. A further study from Finland illustrated that childhood socio-economic class had a very strong relationship with the levels of tooth retention in adulthood [22]. Some authors argue that these findings demonstrate that a more progressive health promotion approach is required, which

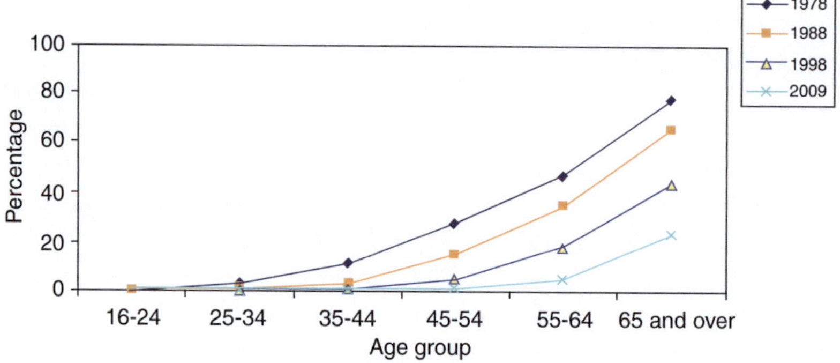

Fig. 4.3 Trends in percentage edentate by age, United Kingdom [17]

recognises the importance of tackling the underlying social, political and environmental determinants of oral health rather than simply treating dental disease and its consequences [23].

4.4.2 The Partially Dentate Older Population

Whilst increasing tooth retention is seen as a significant improvement in the oral health of the older population it does bring with it the emerging challenges of managing chronic dental diseases including caries, periodontal disease and toothwear in older adults. Due to factors such as diet, reduced manual dexterity and xerostomia, these chronic dental diseases can cause considerable pain and suffering amongst older patients and impair oral function.

4.4.3 Dental Caries

Caries can present in older patients as either primary or secondary lesions (Fig. 4.4). Some of the reasons for the development of caries in older adults are a lack of a preventative culture, use of medications that can result in a dry mouth, iatrogenic factors and cognitive and manual dexterity problems which impair oral hygiene [24]. Uptake of dental services by older patients is traditionally low and this may be due to reduced mobility, high cost of dental treatment, negative attitudes or fear of dental procedures and lack of perceived need for oral care. The lack of a preventative culture amongst older adults could also be explained by the fact that, for many years, public oral health promotion programmes were principally aimed at children and adolescents. Older patients were not included in these programmes as their needs were usually perceived as being restricted to the provision of complete replacement dentures.

Primary caries in older adults can present on any tooth surface but it is more commonly seen in cervical areas and on root surfaces. Caries can also develop in susceptible pits and fissures if these have not experienced the disease in the past and therefore have not undergone restoration. Older patients often present with a lifetime of previous dental restorations which may be prone to breakdown and subsequent development of secondary caries. It is known that 60% of restorations placed by practitioners are to replace failed restorations and the most common cause for replacing restorations is secondary caries [25]. Data illustrates that older adults present with high levels of caries [24]. In the 1998 United Kingdom Adult Dental Health Survey, the proportion of adults with 18 or more sound and unrestored teeth was only 5% among those aged 55 years and over [26]. The 2009 United Kingdom Adult Dental Health Survey indicated that this figure had improved but still remained at only 13%. The 2009 United Kingdom Adult Dental Health Survey reported that 27% of adults aged 65–74 years had evidence of caries whilst this figure increased to 40% for those aged 75–84 years [27].

4.4.4 Root Caries

Recession at the gingival margin is a common finding among older patients (Fig. 4.5). As the gingival margin recedes, the cementoenamel junction of the teeth becomes exposed. This is a very irregular site which can be susceptible to bacterial retention and root caries can then develop very quickly. Cementum and dentine on the root are less mineralised than enamel and, as such, are more susceptible to demineralisation. Root caries can present clinically as a spectrum

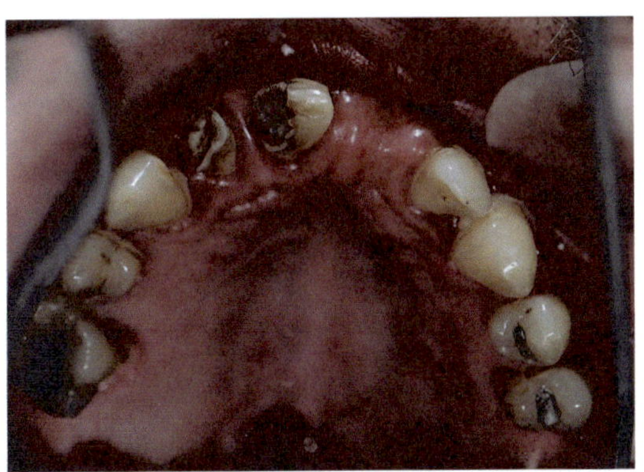

Fig. 4.4 Caries on upper anterior teeth in an older adult

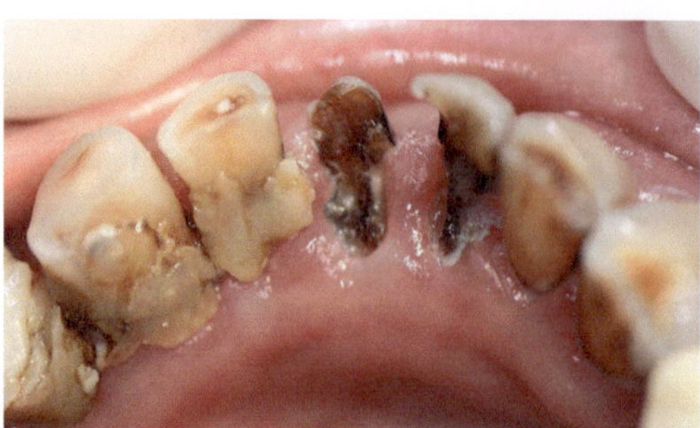

Fig. 4.5 Caries affecting lower anterior teeth

of lesions ranging from very small, softened and discoloured areas to extensive, yellow-brown softened lesions that may encircle the entire root surface [28]. It is important to differentiate between active root caries and arrested lesions in order to plan clinical management. An active lesion is a well-defined, softened area on the root surface that is close to the gingival margin and these lesions are usually covered with plaque. An arrested root surface lesion often appears shiny and hard and is generally further from the gingival margin [14, 29]. Both active and inactive lesions can be cavitated. Active lesions can become arrested if oral hygiene measures are improved, with associated change in texture. Cavitated lesions must be restored if they represent a site of plaque accumulation which results in difficulty in cleaning [30].

The aetiology of dental caries in older adults shares many of the factors described in Chap. 3 in relation to children. Dental caries is fundamentally a multifactorial, bacterially mediated process that results in the destruction of mineralised tooth tissues. A high-sugar-content diet can result in caries with refined carbohydrate fuelling cariogenic bacteria in the mouth. Older patients often consume more cariogenic diets containing large amounts of sugars. Assessing the type and frequency of food intake is important, although proposing changes to older individuals can be quite challenging, particularly for those on restricted diets and those living within residential care. It is essential to know if the diet represents a risk in order to plan the most appropriate treatment and preventive strategy.

The root surface is more vulnerable to mechanical destruction than the enamel due to differences in the structure and chemical composition of cementum and dentine. In a population who are frequently exposed to scaling by dental health professionals, the cementum layer is frequently abraded away, exposing the dentine. Root cementum and dentine are structurally different from enamel and react differently to cariogenic challenges as the critical pH of dentine and cementum is approximately 6.4 whilst that of enamel is 5.5 [28]. Systemic comorbidities, including arthritis or Parkinson's disease, may impair manual dexterity making oral hygiene maintenance a significant challenge in older adults. As older adults lose independence, they may need assistance in performing oral hygiene tasks from a carer or family member. Saliva is essential to keep the mouth relatively clean as it washes away food debris and provides a buffering effect against cariogenic challenges. Therefore, xerostomia is a significant risk factor for development of caries. Unfortunately some dental interventions may also contribute to the process with poorly designed fixed and removable prostheses acting as plaque-retentive elements in the mouth [13].

Older adults present with a unique set of aetiological factors which make them vulnerable to the development of root caries. The 1998 United Kingdom Dental Health Survey showed that almost 25% of older adults had 12 or more teeth with a root surface that was either exposed, worn, filled or decayed [26]. The 2009 Survey reported that 73% of all adults had exposed root surfaces and this increased to 90% for those aged over 55 years. The same survey reported that 11% of 55–64-year-olds had active root caries compared with 20% of those aged 75–84 years [27].

4.4.5 Periodontal Disease

Periodontal disease is a broad term used to describe a range of conditions which impact the supporting structures around the natural teeth. Periodontal disease is considered a chronic dental disease. Although age alone is not considered an independent risk factor for disease development the increased prevalence of periodontal disease in older adults represents a lifetime of periodontal breakdown [31]. For many older patients this presents as gingival recession, thus leaving the exposed root surfaces vulnerable to caries.

It is well established that periodontal disease has modifiable and non-modifiable risk factors which need to be identified as part of any treatment plan when managing older patients [32]. The relationship between smoking and periodontal disease is well established with smoking impairing healing of the periodontal tissues. A number of chronic systemic diseases are regarded as risk factors for periodontal disease including diabetes, cardiovascular disease and dementia [33–35]. Whilst diabetes has a well-established bidirectional relationship with periodontal disease the links with cognitive decline are less well described at this time. Systemic diseases including dementia may impact the ultimate goal of periodontal treatment which is to optimise oral hygiene behaviours and remove plaque-retentive factors, thus encouraging healing of the tissues. A patient's ability to carry out their oral care independently should be considered. If patients are no longer able to carry out their own oral hygiene routine, they become reliant on caregivers to ensure maintenance of their oral hygiene. Older individuals may not cooperate with toothbrushing from caregivers who may not have been trained in how to deliver effective oral care [36]. Aggression, refusing oral care or abusive language is more common in older adults who are cognitively impaired. If adequate toothbrushing is not possible, it is reasonable to explore alternative options such as the use of mouthwashes and sponges; however, it is worth noting that the evidence for the effectiveness of chlorhexidine in reducing dental plaque is only if it is used as an adjunct, rather than an alternative to brushing [37].

Adherence to healthy lifestyle factors has been shown to reduce patients' risk of periodontal disease progression and tooth loss, whereas patients who are overweight or obese have been shown to have an increased risk of periodontitis [38, 39]. The Consensus Statement from the Seventh European Workshop on Periodontology emphasised the importance of giving nutritional advice as part of primary prevention and this topic is discussed in Chap. 6 [40].

4.4.6 Toothwear

Toothwear is a chronic dental disease where tooth substance is gradually lost due to repetitive physical contacts or chemical dissolution (Fig. 4.6). It can be caused by abrasion, attrition or erosion. The most common type of toothwear in older patients is physiological and all dentate older patients will manifest some degree of toothwear. There are four types of toothwear: *Physiological* toothwear is the loss of tooth structure associated with ageing with no associated pathology. *Abrasion* is due to extrinsic physical forces. *Attrition* is due to intrinsic physical forces. *Erosion* is due to the action of acids on the teeth [41].

With increasing age, levels of toothwear increase. Toothwear in older adults is a reflection of a lifetime's exposure to physiological and pathological influences. Physiological toothwear is the normal toothwear which is associated with normal day-to-day functioning. Toothwear can be described as pathological if the remaining tooth structure or pulpal health is compromised, or when the rate of toothwear is in excess of what

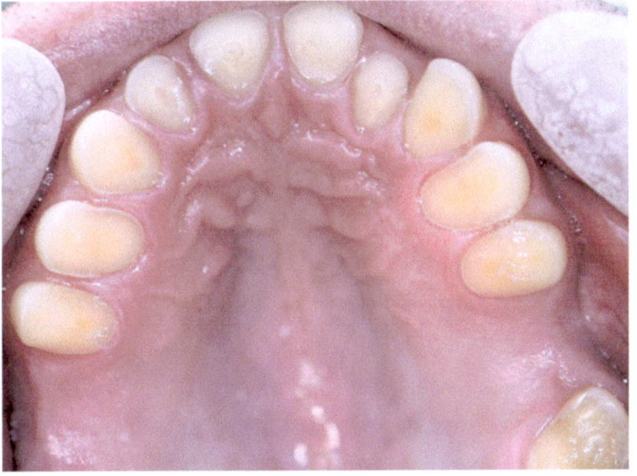

Fig. 4.6 Clinical presentation of toothwear on upper teeth

would be expected for that age. Toothwear can also be considered to be pathological if the patient experiences a deficit as a result of the toothwear in terms of aesthetics or masticatory ability. To put matters in perspective, many older people have significant toothwear but may not have felt the need for treatment [42, 43].

Whilst most toothwear will present with a multifactorial aetiology, erosive toothwear can be caused by either intrinsic or extrinsic sources of acid entering the mouth. Intrinsic sources of acid include gastrointestinal reflux (GERD) and hiatus hernia [44, 45]. However, extrinsic sources are often dietary in nature including consumption of large amounts of citrus fruits, fruit juices, vinegar and some alcoholic beverages. Erosion can appear as loss of tooth structure on the labial or palatal surfaces. Usually, if the source of erosion is extrinsic, the toothwear will appear on the labial surface. Erosion appears on the palatal surface if the source of acid is intrinsic or if there is a distinct pattern of consumption of extrinsic acids. Erosion is characterised by a shiny, glassy appearance with rounded edges, in contrast to the sharp edges associated with abrasion [46]. Whilst tooth tissue may be lost, existing restorations, such as amalgam, are unaffected so that they may project from the surface of the tooth. There may also be a reduced vertical dimension or absence of staining on the teeth, which would occur due to the cleaning effect of the acid [41].

Most older dentate patients have toothwear but there is not a compelling need to treat all toothwear in this population. Treatment is justified if the patient has symptoms such as sensitivity, pulpitis or sharp edges of tooth tissue that are traumatising the soft tissues. Treatment is also warranted when the toothwear has compromised the remaining tooth, so that further loss of tooth tissue would lead to weakening and undermining of the tooth. Another condition demanding treatment is when the patient has a functional deficit—the extent of toothwear is such that the patient has difficulty masticating or he/she has concerns about the aesthetic appearance of his/her teeth. It is not uncommon for family members to encourage older patients with toothwear to see treatment for aesthetic reasons. Providing operative treatment for older adults with toothwear can be challenging and may involve a combination of adhesive dentistry with fixed and removable prosthodontics depending on the clinical presentation and treatment plan [47–49]. However, operative care should not proceed without a preventative programme focused on reducing or eliminating the underlying aetiology including erosive foods and beverages within the diet.

4.5 Conclusion

Evolving population dynamics are already having significant impacts on many aspects of society including healthcare, social policy and economy. In addition to an ageing population we have also seen the emergence of a partially dentate older population with increasing numbers of older adults retaining natural teeth into old age. These changes bring challenges for oral healthcare as preventing and managing chronic dental diseases including caries, periodontal disease and toothwear take on increased importance. In many countries this may necessitate a redesigning of existing delivery models and imaginative workforce planning as outdated systems no longer meet the needs of dentate older adults.

Acknowledgement Figures 4.1 and 4.2 have been reproduced from the World Population Ageing by the Department of Economic Social Affairs Population Division, © 2015 United Nations. Reprinted with the permission of the United Nations.

Figure 4.3 has been reproduced using information from NHS Digital, licenced under the current version of the Open Government Licence.

References

1. Lesthaeghe R, Moors G. Europe's demographic issues: fertility, household formation and replacement migration. United Nations Expert Group Meeting on Policy Responses to Population Decline and Ageing, New York, October 16–18, 2000, UN Population Division; reprinted by the Netherlands Society for International Affairs in: Population Issues—The Human Dimension, 2000. p. 45–73.
2. United Nations. United Nations Department of Economic and Social Affairs, Population Division

Department of Economic and Social Affairs, Population Division. World Population Ageing. 2015.

3. López-Campos JL, Tan W, Soriano JB. Global burden of COPD. Respirology. 2016;21(1):14–23. https://doi.org/10.1111/resp.12660.

4. Farrar NS. With respect to old age: long term care-rights and responsibilities. Br J Soc Work. 2000;30(6):897–9.

5. Boss GR, Seegmiller JE. Age-related physiological changes and their clinical significance. West J Med. 1981;135(6):434–40.

6. Roberts S, Colombier P, Sowman A, et al. Ageing in the musculoskeletal system. Acta Orthop. 2016;87:15–25. https://doi.org/10.1080/17453674.2016.1244750.

7. Pati S, Agrawal S, Swain S, et al. Non communicable disease multimorbidity and associated health care utilization and expenditures in India: cross-sectional study. BMC Health Serv Res. 2014;14:451. https://doi.org/10.1186/1472-6963-14-451.

8. Barnett K, Mercer SW, Norbury M, Watt G, Wyke S, Guthrie B. Epidemiology of multimorbidity and implications for health care, research, and medical education: a cross-sectional study. Lancet. 2012;380(9836):37–43. https://doi.org/10.1016/S0140-6736(12)60240-2.

9. Wallace E, Salisbury C, Guthrie B, Lewis C, Fahey T, Smith SM. Managing patients with multimorbidity in primary care. BMJ. 2015;350:h176. https://doi.org/10.1136/bmj.h176.

10. Raghupathi W, Raghupathi V. An empirical study of chronic diseases in the United States: a visual analytics approach. Int J Environ Res Public Health. 2018;15(3):431. https://doi.org/10.3390/ijerph15030431.

11. World Health Organization. Noncommunicable diseases country profiles 2018. Geneva, Switzerland: World Health Organization; 2018.

12. Wiener RC, Wu B, Crout R, et al. Hyposalivation and xerostomia in dentate older adults. J Am Dent Assoc. 2010;141(3):279–84. https://doi.org/10.14219/jada.archive.2010.0161.

13. Hayes M, Da Mata C, Cole M, McKenna G, Burke F, Allen PF. Risk indicators associated with root caries in independently living older adults. J Dent. 2016;51:8–14. https://doi.org/10.1016/j.jdent.2016.05.006.

14. Hayes M, Allen E, Da Mata C, McKenna G, Burke F. Minimal intervention dentistry and older patients Part 1: Risk assessment and caries prevention. Dent Update. 2014;41(5):406–8. https://doi.org/10.12968/denu.2014.41.5.406.

15. Matear DW, Locker D, Stephens M, Lawrence HP. Associations between xerostomia and health status indicators in the elderly. J R Soc Promot Heal. 2006;126(2):79–85. https://doi.org/10.1177/1466424006063183.

16. Prince M, Bryce R, Albanese E, Wimo A, Ribeiro W, Ferri CP. The global prevalence of dementia: a systematic review and meta-analysis. Alzheimer's Dement. 2013;9(1):63–75. https://doi.org/10.1016/j.jalz.2012.11.007.

17. Steele J, Sullivan IO. Executive summary: adult dental health survey 2009. Heal San Francisco. 2011.

18. Guiney H, Woods N, Whelton H, O'Mullane D. Non-biological factors associated with tooth retention in Irish adults. Commun Dent Health. 2011;28(1):53–9. https://doi.org/10.1922/CDH_2523Guiney07.

19. Cronin M, Meaney S, Jepson NJA, Allen PF. A qualitative study of trends in patient preferences for the management of the partially dentate state. Gerodontology. 2009;26(2):137–42. https://doi.org/10.1111/j.1741-2358.2008.00239.x.

20. Pearce MS, Thomson WM, Walls AWG, Steele JG. Lifecourse socio-economic mobility and oral health in middle age. J Dent Res. 2009;88(10):938–41. https://doi.org/10.1177/0022034509344524.

21. Aida J, Kondo K, Kondo N, Watt RG, Sheiham A, Tsakos G. Income inequality, social capital and self-rated health and dental status in older Japanese. Soc Sci Med. 2011;73(10):1561–8. https://doi.org/10.1016/j.socscimed.2011.09.005.

22. Bernabé E, Watt RG, Sheiham A, et al. Childhood socioeconomic position, adult sense of coherence and tooth retention. Community Dent Oral Epidemiol. 2012;40(1):46–52. https://doi.org/10.1111/j.1600-0528.2011.00633.x.

23. Sheiham A. Delivering dental care: changing needs and future requirements. Br Dent J. 2005;199:187. https://doi.org/10.1038/sj.bdj.4812682.

24. Da Mata C, McKenna G, Burke FM. Caries and the older patient. Dent Update. 2011;38(6):376 8. https://doi.org/10.12968/denu.2011.38.6.376.

25. Javidi H, Tickle M, Aggarwal VR. Repair vs. replacement of failed restorations in general dental practice: Factors influencing treatment choices and outcomes. Br Dent J. 2015;218(1):E2. https://doi.org/10.1038/sj.bdj.2014.1165.

26. Kelly M, Steele J, Nuttall N, Bradnock G, Morris J, Nunn J, et al. Adult dental health survey: oral health in the United Kingdom 1998. London: Palgrave Macmillan; 1998.

27. White DA, Tsakos G, Pitts NB, et al. Adult dental health survey 2009: common oral health conditions and their impact on the population. Br Dent J. 2012;213(11):567–72. https://doi.org/10.1038/sj.bdj.2012.1088.

28. Hayes M, Blum IR, da Mata C. Contemporary challenges and management of dental caries in the older population. Prim Dent J. 2020;9(3):18–22. https://doi.org/10.1177/2050168420943075.

29. Hayes M, Allen E, Da Mata C, McKenna G, Burke F. Minimal intervention dentistry and older patients Part 2: minimally invasive operative interventions. Dent Update. 2014;41(6):500–2. https://doi.org/10.12968/denu.2014.41.6.500.

30. Da Mata C, McKenna G, Anweigi L, et al. An RCT of atraumatic restorative treatment for older adults: 5 year results. J Dent. 2019;83:95–9. https://doi.org/10.1016/j.jdent.2019.03.003.

31. Renvert S, Persson GR. Treatment of periodontal disease in older adults. Periodontol2000. 2016;72(1):108–19. https://doi.org/10.1111/prd.12130.

32. Genco RJ, Borgnakke WS. Risk factors for periodontal disease. Periodontol 2000. 2013;62(1):59–94. https://doi.org/10.1111/j.1600-0757.2012.00457.x.

33. Briggs JE, McKeown PP, Crawford VLS, et al. Angiographically confirmed coronary heart disease and periodontal disease in middle-aged males. J Periodontol. 2006;77(1):95–102. https://doi.org/10.1902/jop.2006.77.1.95.

34. Linden GJ, Lyons A, Scannapieco FA. Periodontal systemic associations: review of the evidence. J Clin Periodontol. 2013;40:S8–S19. https://doi.org/10.1111/jcpe.12064.

35. Tonetti MS, Aiuto FD, Nibali L, et al. Treatment of periodontitis and endothelial function. New Engl J Med. 2007;356(9):911–20.

36. Graham L, Turner W. Periodontal Disease in an Ageing Population: Key Considerations in Diagnosis and Management for the Dental Healthcare Professional. Prim Dent J. 2020;9(3):23–8. https://doi.org/10.1177/2050168420943407.

37. James P, Worthington HV, Parnell C, et al. Chlorhexidine mouthrinse as an adjunctive treatment for gingival health. Cochrane Database Syst Rev. 2017;3(3):CD008676. https://doi.org/10.1002/14651858.CD008676.pub2.

38. Iwasaki M, Borgnakke WS, Ogawa H, et al. Effect of lifestyle on 6-year periodontitis incidence or progression and tooth loss in older adults. J Clin Periodontol. 2018;45(8):896–908. https://doi.org/10.1111/jcpe.12920.

39. Martinez-Herrera M, Silvestre-Rangil J, Silvestre FJ. Association between obesity and periodontal disease: A systematic review of epidemiological studies and controlled clinical trials. Med Oral Patol Oral Cir Bucal. 2017;22(6):e708–15. https://doi.org/10.4317/medoral.21786.

40. Sanz M, Lang NP, Kinane DF, Berglundh T, Chapple I, Tonetti MS. Seventh European Workshop on Periodontology of the European Academy of Periodontology at the Parador at La Granja, Segovia. Spain J Clin Periodontol. 2011;38:1–2. https://doi.org/10.1111/j.1600-051X.2010.01692.x.

41. Burke FM, McKenna G. Toothwear and the older patient. Dent Update. 2011;38(3):165–8. https://doi.org/10.12968/denu.2011.38.3.165.

42. Gilmour AG, Morgan CL. Restorative management of the elderly patient. Prim Dent Care. 2003;10(2):45–8. https://doi.org/10.1308/135576103322500728.

43. Allen F. Pragmatic care for an aging compromised dentition. Aust Dent J. 2019;64(S1):S63–70. https://doi.org/10.1111/adj.12670.

44. Jordão HWT, Coleman HG, Kunzmann AT, McKenna G. The association between erosive toothwear and gastro-oesophageal reflux-related symptoms and disease: a systematic review and meta-analysis. J Dent. 2020;95:103284. https://doi.org/10.1016/j.jdent.2020.103284.

45. Jordão HWT, McKenna G, McMenamin ÚC, Kunzmann AT, Murray LJ, Coleman HG. The association between self-reported poor oral health and gastrointestinal cancer risk in the UK Biobank: A large prospective cohort study. United Eur Gastroenterol J. 2019;7(9):1241–9. https://doi.org/10.1177/2050640619858043.

46. O'Toole S, Bernabé E, Moazzez R, Bartlett D. Timing of dietary acid intake and erosive tooth wear: a case-control study. J Dent. 2017;56:99–104. https://doi.org/10.1016/j.jdent.2016.11.005.

47. Allen PF. Use of tooth-coloured restorations in the management of toothwear. Dent Update. 2003;30(10):550–6. https://doi.org/10.12968/denu.2003.30.10.550.

48. Yule PL, Barclay SC. Worn down by toothwear? Aetiology, diagnosis and management revisited. Dent Update. 2015;42(6):525–6. https://doi.org/10.12968/denu.2015.42.6.525.

49. Al-Khayatt AS, Ray-Chaudhuri A, Poyser NJ, et al. Direct composite restorations for the worn mandibular anterior dentition: A 7-year follow-up of a prospective randomised controlled split-mouth clinical trial. J Oral Rehabil. 2013;40(5):389–401. https://doi.org/10.1111/joor.12042.

The Importance of Nutrition for Older Adults

5

Jayne V. Woodside, Sara M. Wallace, Michelle C. McKinley, Anne P. Nugent, and Gerry McKenna

Abstract

A key public health issue is the health of the increasing global ageing population. Such a population shift will necessitate changes and improvements to healthcare systems and individual lifestyle behaviours to ensure that adults who are living longer are doing so in good health. Just as in any other age group, adequate nutrition is paramount to ensure optimal physical and mental functioning for older adults. However, the ability to achieve adequate nutritional status will be affected by a range of factors; for example chronic illnesses can have a direct impact on nutritional status, while suffering from poor mental health can affect appetite.

J. V. Woodside (✉) · S. M. Wallace · M. C. McKinley
The Institute for Global Food Security, School of Biological Sciences, Queen's University Belfast, Belfast, United Kingdom

Centre for Public Health, School of Medicine, Dentistry and Biomedical Sciences, Queen's University Belfast, Belfast, United Kingdom
e-mail: j.woodside@qub.ac.uk

A. P. Nugent
The Institute for Global Food Security, School of Biological Sciences, Queen's University Belfast, Belfast, United Kingdom

Institute of Food and Health, University College Dublin, Dublin, Ireland

G. McKenna
Centre for Public Health, School of Medicine, Dentistry and Biomedical Sciences, Queen's University Belfast, Belfast, United Kingdom

This chapter aims to describe the ageing population and nutritional requirements of older adults, present the evidence linking nutrition and chronic disease risk and then summarise the factors that affect dietary intake, nutritional status and malnutrition risk of older adults, including medical, physical, psychological, social and economic factors, which can have both direct and indirect impact on dietary intake.

5.1 Nutrition and Ageing

For older people, who are at increased risk of chronic disease, eating a healthy, balanced diet, ideally starting from a young age, can help to decrease the incidence and progression of disease and promote long-term healthy, independent living [1, 2]. However, the ageing process is accompanied by various changes which can impair the ability to eat well, resulting in a decrease in appetite and food intake as well as diet quality [3, 4].

5.1.1 Dietary Recommendations and Guidelines for Older Adults

Dietary recommendations for older adults differ by global region. The Academy of Nutrition and Dietetics recommends that older adults consume the same diets as adults in general, as per the Dietary Guidelines for Americans, including eating fruits and vegetables, varied protein sources and three servings of dairy products per day, with no specific nutrient recommendations for this age group [5]. In contrast, the Department of Health in the United Kingdom has different nutrient intake guidelines for older adults, recommending slightly lower intakes of energy, fat and carbohydrates; slightly higher intakes of protein for females; and similar intakes of dietary fibre and micronutrients compared to the younger population [6]. Food-based guidelines are, however, similar across all ages [7]. Countries such as Australia appear to make more specific recommendations for older adults in their dietary guidelines, stating that "older people should eat nutritious foods and keep physically active to help maintain muscle strength and a healthy weight" [8]. This separation is also seen in the joint nutrient reference values for Australia and New Zealand, with slightly higher intakes recommended of protein and riboflavin for those aged over 70 and higher intake of vitamin B6 for women over 50 [9].

5.1.2 Dietary Intake in Older Adults

As people age, there is a well-recognised linear decrease in food intake [10]. Between the ages of approximately 20 and 80, total energy intake can decrease by as much as 800 kcal and 1000 kcal in men and women, respectively [11].

According to the National Diet and Nutrition Survey, older adults in the United Kingdom are not consuming the recommended number of kcal per day, or portions of fruits, vegetables and oily fish, and men aged 65 years and older exceeded the recommendation for red and processed meat consumption [12, 13]. It was also observed that a substantial proportion of older adults in the United Kingdom were consuming intakes below the lower reference nutrient intake for micronutrients such as selenium and vitamin D. Similarly, a systematic review conducted in 2015 observed a high prevalence of a number of micronutrient inadequacies amongst community-dwelling older adults, in particular thiamin, riboflavin, vitamin D, calcium, magnesium and selenium [14].

5.1.3 Malnutrition

Malnutrition is defined as a "state of nutrition in which a deficiency or excess (or imbalance) of energy, protein and other nutrients causes measurable adverse effects on tissue/body for (body shape, size and composition) and function and clinical outcome" and is a serious multifactorial issue for the older adult population [15]. This definition is broad and therefore encompasses both under- and overnutrition; however, in the older population the term malnutrition is usually considered as undernutrition. Evidence suggests that nearly one-third of older patients are classed as at risk of malnutrition upon hospital admission, and patients with malnutrition had a 3-day longer hospital stay compared to well-nourished individuals, as well as saw their GP twice as often and got admitted to hospital three times more often [16]. Within the care home setting, the prevalence of malnutrition can reach up to 45% in some areas of the United Kingdom. There are many consequences of malnutrition in older people, including poorer quality of life, greater susceptibility to infection and increased morbidity and mortality [17–19].

One way to reduce the burden of malnutrition in older people, particularly in clinical settings, is through the use of oral nutrition support (ONS), which, in the United Kingdom, is recommended for individuals with a "Body Mass Index of less than 18.5 kg/m^2 or unintentional weight loss greater than 10% within the last 3–6 months" [20]. The National Institute for Health and Care Excellence (NICE) has estimated that, if the treatment and detection of malnutrition were improved according to NICE guidance, there would be likely annual cost savings of £45.5 million, and an economic analysis estimated annual savings of approximately £90,000 from reductions in length of hospital stays through the efficient use of ONS [21, 22].

5.1.4 Obesity

New evidence from the United States has demonstrated a shift towards obesity and higher calorie and fat diets amongst the older population, as well as higher waist circumferences and waist-to-hip ratios when compared to younger adults [23–25]. Protective effects of obesity in older age include increased bone mineral density and decreased risk of developing osteoporosis and hip fractures [26]. However, these positive effects are greatly outweighed by the many negative effects of obesity on health and well-being in older age, including a decrease in physical functioning, reduced quality of life and increased risk of chronic diseases [27–29]. It has also been observed that although obese individuals consume higher-than-recommended calorie intakes, they also display higher rates of micronutrient deficiencies than those who are not obese.

5.1.5 Reduced Dietary Variety

Dietary variety (DV), as defined by Maslin et al. in 2016, is the "number of different foods or food groups consumed over a given reference period" that is positively associated with dietary quality [30]. Globally, older adults have been shown to have a reduced DV, which is concerning, as DV has been associated with a reduced risk of several chronic diseases and utilisation of healthcare services [31–34].

5.2 Diet and Chronic Disease Risk in Older Age

As the following sections demonstrate, poor nutritional intake and status have been associated with increased risk of a range of chronic diseases, while being in ill health also affects the ability and desire to eat, and consequent dietary intake [35]. As the population ages, the prevalence and associated burden of chronic diseases are projected to increase, placing the affected individuals at a greater risk of impaired nutritional status and malnutrition-related health issues. Therefore, optimising dietary intake in older populations has the potential to reduce the risk of chronic disease.

5.2.1 Cancer

Evidence-based World Cancer Research Fund Cancer Prevention Recommendations, supported by systematic reviews which are regularly updated, state that, alongside avoiding tobacco exposure and excess sun, making dietary changes such as limiting consumption of red and processed meat and eating a diet rich in fruits, vegetables, beans and wholegrains is associated with reduced risk of cancer [36]. The 2018 World Cancer Research Fund Expert Report has highlighted strong evidence that exposure to dairy products, wholegrains and foods containing dietary fibre is associated with decreased risk of colorectal cancer, and risk of cancers of the aerodigestive tract, including some head and neck cancers, is associated with increased consumption of non-starchy vegetables and fruits [37]. Furthermore, the risk of developing colorectal cancer has been associated with increased consumption of red and processed meat, and consuming diets with a greater glycaemic load has been associated with increased risk of endometrial cancer [38]. The risk of developing colorectal cancer, as well as cancers of the oesophagus, pancreas, liver, breast and endometrium, is associated with increased adult body fatness and being obese or overweight throughout adulthood [39].

Post-diagnosis and during treatment, appetite, energy intake and nutritional status can be considerably impaired, and malnutrition is common in cancer patients, with many experiencing significant weight loss during progression of the disease [40]. The physical and emotional effects of chemotherapy treatments, as well as obstructions caused by tumours, can affect taste, smell and appetite and produce sore mouth, nausea, vomiting, diarrhoea and constipation, all of which can contribute to poor food intake and nutrient malabsorption [41]. An extreme form of anorexia, cachexia, can occur in some cancer patients and is characterised by a weight loss of at least 5% within a year or less in the presence of underlying cancer, and an additional three criteria, including decreased muscle strength, fatigue, anorexia, low fat-free mass index and atypical biochemistry [42]. ONS may be required if malnutrition and weight loss are severe.

5.2.2 Cardiovascular Disease

Systematic reviews have identified causal associations between coronary heart disease and intakes of a range of foods and nutrients including monounsaturated and trans-fatty acids, nuts, foods with a high glycaemic index, as well as overall dietary quality and dietary patterns [43, 44]. Whole-diet approaches, such as Mediterranean-style diets, high in fruits, vegetables, fish, olive oil and legumes and low in red meat and other processed foods, have been shown to improve cardiovascular risk factors such as weight gain and blood pressure, and randomised trials with hard clinical endpoints have confirmed the efficacy of this diet pattern [45, 46].

5.2.3 Respiratory Diseases

Respiratory conditions, such as chronic obstructive pulmonary disease (COPD), have been shown to be associated with ageing, with the prevalence of COPD increasing up to threefold in individuals over the age of 60 [47]. COPD has been observed to affect nutritional status by a variety of mechanisms, including energy imbalance, primarily due to increased energy required for breathing, atrophy of the muscles due to reduced physical function, hypoxaemia, systemic inflammation, oxidative stress and hypogonadism in some patients [48, 49]. Although in high-income countries smoking cigarettes is the main risk factor for respiratory diseases such as COPD, diet has also been shown to influence risk. Data from a 2016 systematic review observed associations between dietary patterns and risk of COPD, with individuals following more Western-type dietary patterns having an increased risk and individuals following a prudent dietary pattern (high in fruits, vegetables, fish and wholegrains) having a reduced risk of newly diagnosed COPD [50].

5.2.4 Osteoporosis

Osteoporosis is characterised by reduced bone mineral density, increased brittleness and fragility of bones, and increased risk of fractures. Prevalence rates are higher in older people, and the condition is more common in women than in men. There is evidence to suggest that adults, particularly postmenopausal women, are not consuming adequate levels of calcium as part of their diet; therefore it is recommended by NICE and the National Osteoporosis Guideline Group that adults should consume a daily intake of between 700 and 1200 mg of calcium per day to improve bone health [51]. Calcium supplementation is recommended if dietary intake is below 700 mg/day amongst postmenopausal women and older men receiving osteoporotic treatment, such as bisphosphonates and calcitonin. Vitamin D supplementation (800 IU/day of cholecalciferol) is also advised for this population group and for those at risk of vitamin D insufficiency [51].

There is also evidence to suggest a beneficial role of other micronutrients, such as vitamin K and potassium. These micronutrients can be found in the diet in the form of fruits and vegetables, and those consuming higher levels of vitamin K and potassium have been shown to have a lower incidence of bone fractures, higher BMD and less bone loss [52, 53].

5.2.5 Frailty

A recent consensus report on frailty defined the condition as "a medical syndrome with multiple causes and contributors that is characterized by diminished strength, endurance, and reduced physiologic function that increases an individual's vulnerability for developing increased dependency and/or death" [54]. Frailty has been found to be an independent predictor of risk of adverse outcomes, including falls, hospitalisation, disability and death, and can affect up to 59% and 80% of older adults in the community and secondary care, respectively [54, 55]. The development of frailty can be attributed to a combination of factors, such as reduced food intake, sarcopenia, chronic disease, cachexia, malnutrition and impaired functional ability [56]. Higher intakes of total protein combined with exercise have been associated with a reduced risk of frailty, particularly when compared to individual amino acid intake [57]. There is evidence to suggest that increasing protein intake, combined with a diet high in calcium and vitamin D, can enhance bone and muscle health, as well as reduce fall and fracture risk in frail older adult populations [58]. Several systematic reviews have noted the influence of malnutrition on frailty in the older adult population; therefore oral nutritional supplements (ONS) and other means of enteral nutrition have been recommended as treatment for frail older adults at risk of malnutrition in an attempt to reduce mortality, and improve nutritional status, quality of life and functional ability [59–61].

5.2.6 Sarcopenia

While frailty is a medical syndrome characterised by diminished strength and endurance, sarcopenia is characterised by a progressive and generalised loss of skeletal muscle mass and strength [62]. Sarcopenia has been shown to be a prominent cause of frailty, impaired functional ability and nutritional status in older people [63]. Prevalence of sarcopenia appears to vary according to country, but overall prevalence has been estimated to be 10% amongst community-dwelling adults aged over 60 years [64]. As for frailty, certain micronutrients (folic acid, vitamin B6 and magnesium) and macronutrients (protein) have been suggested as playing a prominent role in the risk of sarcopenia. Research suggests that dietary sources of protein were inversely associated with loss of lean muscle mass in older adults and suggested that interventions to encourage the consumption of protein to a level higher than currently recommended may reduce the loss of lean mass that occurs in ageing [65]. Recent research has found that factors such as the maintenance of a healthy body weight and taking part in resistance exercise, along with adequate or enhanced intakes of vitamin D, amino acids such as leucine

and protein, could reduce the burden of sarcopenia in older adults and improve bone density, muscle strength and mass [66]. Similar results were obtained from a 2012 review conducted in the USA, and there is a large body of literature suggesting that utilising amino acids to improve protein synthesis in ageing muscle is a potential target for intervention development for sarcopenia in the global older adult population [67–70].

Sarcopenic obesity can, however, also occur in old age, due to increasing obesity rates in older adults. This condition is characterised by high levels of fat mass and low levels of muscle mass, and is associated with functional decline and increased risk of morbidity and disability [71].

5.2.7 Parkinson's Disease

Conditions such as Parkinson's disease can affect food intake, since movement and hand-mouth coordination can be difficult. Capability to shop, cook and feed independently may also be impaired, and this may explain patients with Parkinson's having a lower BMI when compared to healthy subjects, as well as an altered distribution of body fat [72]. A 2014 review conducted in the USA noted that, although there is a plethora of preliminary evidence to suggest the role of nutrition in the development and prevention of Parkinson's disease, mainly focussing on oxidative stress, further research needs to be conducted in the area to develop the evidence base, particularly if this is to become an avenue for potential treatment options [73].

5.2.8 Dementia

A range of nutritional factors have been associated with reduced risk of cognitive decline. Obesity in adulthood has been demonstrated to be a risk factor for dementia and cognitive impairment in older age [74]. However, issues surrounding food intake and behaviour can vary throughout the progression of dementia. In the initial stages, the patient can overeat, and, as the disease progresses, the patient may have difficulty eating and even refuse to eat. In the later stages, the patient may require help with feeding, as they are unable to feed themselves. It is common to see dementia patients lose a substantial amount of body weight in the later stages of the disease. Individuals with dementia have also been found to be more likely to practice unsafe food storage and handling practices, placing them at an increased risk of food-borne illness [75, 76].

Screening to identify malnutrition in dementia patients is vital, and, in care homes and hospitals, staff members and volunteers should be trained in providing feeding assistance to all patients, but in particular those with dementia, to help improve food intake. Eating with people who are familiar, encouragement by carers, patient choice in meals and modifying eating environments to ensure a more enjoyable eating experience can also help to improve food intake [77]. If these methods are unsuccessful, ONS or enteral nutrition may be required in those who are severely malnourished.

5.3 Factors Affecting Diet and Nutritional Status in Older Adults

There are a wide range of complex factors which can affect an older person's diet and can lead to reduced diet quality and potentially malnutrition. Each of these factors needs to be taken into consideration when examining diet in older people and encouraging eating behaviours that will promote healthy ageing. Oral health, including retention or replacement of natural teeth, is an important factor influencing diet in older adults but this will be discussed in detail in Chap. 7.

5.3.1 Appetite and Satiety

As previously discussed, older adults consume fewer calories from meals and snacks, and have poorer appetites and are more easily satisfied post-meal consumption, potentially due to slower gastric emptying [78]. Such lower levels of appetite can also impair diet quality and variety [79].

5.3.2 Food Safety and Hygiene Practices

As people age, they are at a much greater risk of contracting food-borne illnesses and infections and dying from such infections. A report from the WHO suggests that adults >60 were 2.6 times more susceptible to developing serious illness from consuming the pathogen *Listeria monocytogenes* compared to the general population. This increased risk is due to a variety of reasons, including a decrease in the functioning of the immune system, co-occurrence of chronic diseases and potential nutrient deficiency such as vitamin C, iron and folic acid [80–82]. Of concern, food safety practices in older people in the United Kingdom may be less stringent, with up to 66% reporting consuming foods beyond the recommended 2 days after opening. Other unsafe food storage and handling practices were reported, including unsafe refrigeration temperatures and not keeping raw and cooked meats separated [83]. These issues were magnified in older adults suffering from dementia or cognitive decline, and also in those who live alone.

5.3.3 Smoking and Alcohol Consumption

Unhealthy behaviours, such as smoking, lack of physical activity, alcohol consumption and poor diet, often cluster within the general population. Globally, in older adults, several smaller studies have noted poorer quality diets being consumed by those who smoke and consume alcohol to excess [84].

5.3.4 Physical Activity

Although research has shown that physical activity can slow down the ageing process in older populations, reduced physical activity levels can often be observed in older people, with as many as 64% of adults aged >65 years not adhering to recommended physical activity guidelines [85]. Reduced levels of physical activity can be due to many reasons, such as avoidance because of pain, fear of falls, increased bed rest, hospitalisation or conditions such as osteoporosis, Parkinson's disease and arthritis. Lower physical activity levels can reduce appetite in older people, since energy expenditure is low, and, therefore, older people may not feel inclined to eat sufficiently for their needs [86]. Recent meta-analyses amongst older adults have shown that exercise may help to increase physical functioning, through improvements in muscle strength and mobility, enhancing the ability to carry out activities of daily living (ADL) [87].

5.3.5 Physical Function

Reduced physical function in older people will affect the ability to go to the supermarket to buy food and to prepare and cook meals. Reduced physical functioning, which can be particularly detrimental in individuals in nursing homes, has also been associated with other health issues, including risk factors for a number of chronic diseases, as well as impairing social interaction and mood. As regular physical activity can help to improve physical functioning in older adults, they should be encouraged by health professionals to incorporate appropriate physical activity where possible into their daily routines [87].

5.3.6 Dysphagia

Dysphagia can also be problematic in older people, with causes including stroke, Parkinson's disease and dementia [88]. Older people with dysphagia are at increased risk of malnutrition and dehydration, with patients reporting lower daily energy intakes than those without dysphagia [89]. As well as physical difficulties, dysphagia and other chewing issues may lead to psychological problems amongst this age group, including anxiety about eating in front of others, leading to avoidance of social eating occasions due to fear or embarrassment [90]. ONS and tube feeding may be required to help attain an adequate intake of nutrients if the patient is unable to swallow a sufficient amount of food or liquid.

5.3.7 Medications

Polypharmacy, which can be defined as "the use of multiple medications and/or the administration of more medications than are clinically indicated", has been identified as a risk factor for malnutrition in older adults, both directly through drug-nutrient interactions and indirectly through effects on appetite [91, 92]. Some medications, such as chemotherapy drugs, can cause nausea and vomiting, therefore increasing the risk of malnutrition; however drugs used to prevent vomiting can also affect nutritional status through dysphagia, taste changes and constipation or diarrhoea. There is evidence to highlight an association between the risk of malnutrition, polypharmacy and drug-nutrient interactions, with older individuals who presented as malnourished being more likely to be taking a higher number of medications compared to well-nourished individuals.

5.3.8 Gastrointestinal Tract Function

Ageing is accompanied by reduced functioning of the gastrointestinal tract. Pernicious anaemia is a particular problem, as the process of vitamin B12 absorption in older adults, involving the stomach, small intestine and pancreas, is less efficient compared to other age groups. It has been observed in up to 70% of cases of older adults with vitamin B12 deficiency that physiological changes render the vitamin B12 unable to be taken up by intrinsic factor for absorption [93].

5.3.9 Sensory Issues

The prevalence of vision impairment, as a result of age-related macular degeneration and cataract, increases greatly with age [94]. Loss in vision can significantly affect the ability of older adults to remain independent, and will affect activities of daily living, such as managing finances, food shopping, reading food labels and preparing and cooking meals. This can negatively affect dietary intake, as some individuals will need to rely on others for the provision of regular, healthy meals.

Hearing loss, which similarly increases with age, has also been associated with poor dietary quality and a reduced ability to perform ADL, such as going to the shops to purchase food, and participating in social activities, such as eating out with family or friends. Furthermore, there is now early evidence to suggest relationships between hearing loss and intakes of certain nutrients such as dietary polyunsaturated fatty acids, vitamin B12 and folate, which, if confirmed, suggests that these modifiable risk factors could be targeted for dietary interventions in this population group [95].

Sense of smell deteriorates with age, potentially due to reduced functioning of olfactory receptors, and so too does the ability to distinguish between different smells. In many cases, loss in taste sensation is in fact due to a deficit in the sense of smell, but Fukanga et al. reported that the taste sensations of sweet, salty, sour and bitter also deteriorate with age, potentially due to medication use and oral health issues [96]. This reduction in taste sensitivity can have a major impact on a person's eating habits, as they lose interest and enjoyment in eating food. Flavour enhancement of food is one method which could help to increase the palatability of food for older people to try to increase their appetite and food intake [97, 98].

5.3.10 Hormonal Status

There is evidence to suggest that hormonal status may have a part to play in reduced dietary intake in older people. Systematic reviews have highlighted the role of gut hormones, including CCK, ghrelin and peptide tyrosine tyrosine (PYY), in the ageing process and their potential effects on satiety, appetite and food intake [99]. The hormone CCK has been found to have a greater satiating effect in older people than in younger people. There is also some evidence to show that both the production and sensitivity of ghrelin and CCK are altered during the ageing process, which may decrease appetite and increase satiety levels

in older people, although research is at an early stage [100].

5.3.11 Depression

Minor depression has been shown to occur frequently in the older adult population, and the condition is under-treated and under-diagnosed in older patients [101]. The causes of depression in old age can be multifactorial, including loneliness, bereavement, boredom or stress, low socioeconomic status, chronic illness, disability and cognitive impairment. Depressed older adults have been shown to have poorer diet quality, including lower intakes of oily fish and fruits and vegetables, and were more likely to be malnourished [102–106]. Furthermore, there is evidence to suggest a bidirectional relationship between food intake and depressive symptoms; it can lead to a loss of interest in food, therefore reducing food intake leading to weight loss, but can also cause increased food intake and obesity [107].

5.3.12 Social Isolation and Loneliness

Social factors, including marital status, loneliness and poverty, have been shown to influence dietary quality and eating habits amongst older adults, and a 2015 meta-analysis reported that these factors may also be associated with mortality risk [108].

Older people who live alone and are socially isolated from others, potentially due to reduced physical function, are inclined to eat less than people who eat in company. Older people are also faced with the loss of loved ones as they get older, and this loss is intensified if there are no children, or if children have moved away. Older adults who have been widowed are more likely to live on their own and may live long distances from their children or family members, and, without encouragement or reminders, may simply forget to eat or find it difficult to adjust to cooking meals for just one person, and are therefore at increased risk of malnutrition [109, 110].

The effect of bereavement on diet has been particularly noted in older men who have recently been widowed, who may lack the skills and knowledge required to cook healthy meals as they may have relied on their partners to cook for them, placing them at an increased risk of consuming a poor diet.

In older adults, particularly in rural areas, a lack of access to transport, particularly amongst those who have recently stopped driving, can result in social isolation, reduced quality of life and reduced ability to obtain a wide variety of healthy, nutritious food when shopping; thus there is potential for the development of interventions to improve public transport and make it more accessible and user friendly for older adults.

5.3.13 Low Income and Socio-Economic Status

The numbers of people experiencing poverty have decreased significantly in recent years; however a lower socio-economic status can still negatively impact health, through influencing diet quality, dietary patterns, food security and nutritional status. Low income can act as a potential barrier to purchasing healthy food, with a significant proportion of older adults reporting that price and money available for food were important factors affecting food choice [111]. A 2013 systematic review noted that older adults were particularly susceptible to displaying a poor nutritional status and reporting reduced food expenditure due to changes in socio-economic situations, namely transitioning from employment to retirement, especially if the retirement was not voluntary [112].

Poverty is seen to be a social determinant of health and ill health, and appears to be closely associated with the level of education, both of which may have a negative impact on health and well-being. Several recent systematic reviews have noted poor health literacy amongst the older adult population [113]. Low levels of health literacy in older adults have been associated with difficulties in understanding health information, therefore making it more difficult to make health-

ier life choices such as participating in physical activity and consuming a healthy diet; however there is little evidence exploring these associations specifically amongst older adults. Globally, a higher prevalence of malnutrition has been observed amongst illiterate older adults, with less educated older adults observed as being least likely to purchase foods high in fibre and low in salt and sugar [114].

5.4 Conclusion

Diet is important to promote good health and reduce chronic disease risk across the life course but, given the fact that our population is ageing, understanding the role of diet in older populations and factors that influence dietary intake is vital. A complex range of factors including medical, physiological, psychological, social and economic factors can influence an older person's diet and lead to poor nutritional status. Consequences of malnutrition in the older adult population include a poorer quality of life, longer hospital stays and increased morbidity and mortality, which contributes to increasing healthcare expenditure, which is unsustainable within an ageing population. Barriers to healthy eating in older people include lack of resources, money, transport, education and limited cooking skills. Therefore, it is important to develop and utilise effective strategies, policies and interventions on both a global and local scale to reduce the burden of chronic disease and improve the quality of life of people in this age group.

References

1. Dean M, Raats MM, Grunert KG, Lumbers M. Factors influencing eating a varied diet in old age. Public Health Nutr. 2009;12(12):2421–7. https://doi.org/10.1017/S1368980009005448.
2. World Health Organisation. Nutrition for older persons. Geneva, Switzerland: World Health Organization.
3. Chapman IM, MacIntosh CG, Morley JE, Horowitz M. The anorexia of ageing. Biogerontology. 2002;3(1-2):67–71.
4. Morley JE. Anorexia of aging: physiologic and pathologic. Am J Clin Nutr. 1997;66:760–73.

5. Nutrition Today. Agriculture USD of H and HS and USD of 2015 – 2020 Dietary Guidelines for Americans. In: 2015 – 2020 Dietary Guidelines for Americans. 8th ed; 2015. p. 18. https://doi.org/10.1097/NT.0b013e31826c50af.

6. Public Health England. Government dietary recommendations. England, UK: Public Health England; 2016. p. 1–12.

7. Public Health England. A quick guide to the government's healthy eating recommendations. England, UK: Public Health England; 2018.

8. National Health and Medical Research Council. Australian Dietary Guidelines (2013). 2013. p. 17–18. https://www.nhmrc.gov.au/guidelines-publications/n55

9. NHMRC Australia. Nutrient Reference Values for Australia and New Zealand Including Recommended Dietary Intakes | National Health and Medical Research Council; 2017.

10. de Boer A, Ter Horst GJ, Lorist MM. Physiological and psychosocial age-related changes associated with reduced food intake in older persons. Ageing Res Rev. 2013;12(1):316–28. https://doi.org/10.1016/j.arr.2012.08.002.

11. Drewnowski A, Evans WJ. Nutrition, physical activity, and quality of life in older adults: summary. J Gerontol. 2001;56(11):89–94.

12. Watson S, McGowan L, McCrum L-A, et al. The impact of dental status on perceived ability to eat certain foods and nutrient intakes in older adults: Cross-sectional analysis of the UK National Diet and Nutrition Survey 2008-2014. Int J Behav Nutr Phys Act. 2019;16(1):43. https://doi.org/10.1186/s12966-019-0803-8.

13. Roberts C, Steer T, Maplethorpe N, et al. National diet and nutrition survey: results from Years 7 and 8 (combined) of the Rolling Programme (2014/2015 - 2015/2016). England, UK: Public Health England; 2018.

14. Ter Borg S, Verlaan S, Hemsworth J, et al. Micronutrient intakes and potential inadequacies of community-dwelling older adults: a systematic review. Br J Nutr. 2015;113(8):1195–206. https://doi.org/10.1017/S0007114515000203.

15. Brotherton A, Cheema K, Holdoway A, Todorovic V, Stroud M. Nutritional care tool report 2017 a report by the BAPEN quality and safety committee nutritional care tool annual report 2017. 2017.

16. Guest JF, Panca M, Baeyens JP, et al. Health economic impact of managing patients following a community-based diagnosis of malnutrition in the UK. Clin Nutr. 2011;30(4):422–9. https://doi.org/10.1016/j.clnu.2011.02.002.

17. Clarke DM, Wahlqvist ML, Strauss BJ. Undereating and undernutrition in old age: integrating bio-psychosocial aspects. Age Ageing. 1998;27(4):527–34.

18. Mountford C, Okonkwo A, HArt K, Thompson N. Managing malnutrition in older persons residing in care homes: nutritional and clinical outcomes following a screening and intervention program. J Nutr Gerontol Geriatr. 2016;35(1):52–66.

19. Forster SE, Powers HJ, Foulds GA, et al. Improvement in nutritional status reduces the clinical impact of infections in older adults. J Am Geriatr Soc. 2012;60(9):1645–54. https://doi.org/10.1111/j.1532-5415.2012.04118.x.

20. National Institute for Health and Care Excellence. Nutrition support for adults: oral nutrition support, enteral tube feeding and parenteral nutrition. London: National Institute for Health and Care Excellence.

21. Wilson L, Health RP. A review and summary of the impact of malnutrition in older people and the reported costs and benefits of interventions. Prev Malnutriotn Later Life. 2013;2013:1–30.

22. Elia M, Zellipour L, Stratton RJ. To screen or not to screen for adult malnutrition? Clin Nutr. 2005;24(6):867–84. https://doi.org/10.1016/j.clnu.2005.03.004.

23. Johnston BC, Kanters S, Bandayrel K, et al. Comparison of weight loss among named diet programs in overweight and obese adults: a meta-analysis. JAMA - J Am Med Assoc. 2014;312(9):923–33. https://doi.org/10.1001/jama.2014.10397.

24. Flegal KM, Kruszon-Moran D, Carroll MD, Fryar CD, Ogden CL. Trends in obesity among adults in the United States, 2005 to 2014. JAMA - J Am Med Assoc. 2016;315(21):2284–91. https://doi.org/10.1001/jama.2016.6458.

25. Fryar C, Carroll M, Ogden C. Prevalence of overweight, obesity, and extreme obesity among adults: United States, trends 1960–1962 through 2009–2010. Natl Cent Heal Stat. 2012;2012:1–8.

26. Villareal DT, Apovian CM, Kushner RF, Klein S. Obesity in older adults: technical review and position statement of the American Society for Nutrition and NAASO, the Obesity Society. Am J Clin Nutr. 2005;82(5):923–34. https://doi.org/10.1038/oby.2005.228.

27. Bowman K, Delgado J, Henley WE, et al. Obesity in older people with and without conditions associated with weight loss: follow-up of 955,000 primary care patients. J Gerontol A Biol Sci Med Sci. 2017;72(2):203–9. https://doi.org/10.1093/gerona/glw147.

28. Corica F, Bianchi G, Corsonello A, Mazzella N, Lattanzio F, Giulio M. Obesity in the context of aging: quality of life considerations. PharmacoEconomics. 2015;33:655–72. https://doi.org/10.1007/s40273-014-0237-8.

29. Kaidar-Person O, Person B, Szomstein S, Rosenthal RJ. Nutritional deficiencies in morbidly obese patients: a new form of malnutrition? Part A: Vitamins. Obes Surg. 2008;18(7):870–6. https://doi.org/10.1007/s11695-007-9349-y.

30. Maslin K, Dean T, Arshad SH, Venter C. Dietary variety and food group consumption in children consuming a cows' milk exclusion diet. Pediatr Allergy Immunol. 2016;27(5):471–7. https://doi.org/10.1111/pai.12573.

31. Conklin AI, Forouhi NG, Suhrcke M, Surtees P, Wareham NJ, Monsivais P. Variety more than quantity of fruit and vegetable intake varies by socioeconomic status and financial hardship. Findings from older adults in the EPIC cohort. Appetite. 2014;83:248–55. https://doi.org/10.1016/j.appet.2014.08.038.

32. Lo Y, Wahlqvist ML, Chang Y, Kao S, Lee M. Dietary diversity predicts type of medical expenditure in elders. Am J Manag Care. 2013;19(12):415–23.

33. Cooper AJ, Sharp SJ, Lentjes MAH, et al. A prospective study of the association between quantity and variety of fruit and vegetable intake and incident type 2 diabetes. Diabetes Care. 2012;35(6):1293–300. https://doi.org/10.2337/dc11-2388.

34. Jeurnink SM, Büchner FL, Bueno-De-Mesquita HB, et al. Variety in vegetable and fruit consumption and the risk of gastric and esophageal cancer in the European prospective investigation into cancer and nutrition. Int J Cancer. 2012;131(6):E963–73. https://doi.org/10.1002/ijc.27517.

35. Lorenzo-López L, Maseda A, De Labra C, Regueiro-Folgueira L, Rodríguez-Villamil JL, Millán-Calenti JC. Nutritional determinants of frailty in older adults: A systematic review. BMC Geriatr. 2017;17(1):108. https://doi.org/10.1186/s12877-017-0496-2.

36. World Cancer Research Fund. Our cancer prevention recommendations. London: World Cancer Research Fund International; last accessed 3rd August 2021.

37. World Cancer Research Fund, Research TAI for C. Continuous Update Project Expert Report 2018. Wholegrains, vegetables and fruit and the risk of cancer. London: World Cancer Research Fund International; 2018.

38. World Cancer Research Fund, Research TAI for C. Continuous update project expert report 2018. Other dietary exposures and the risk of cancer. London: World Cancer Research Fund International; 2018.

39. World Cancer Research Fund, Research TAI for C. Continuous Update Project Expert Report 2018. Body fatness and weight gain and the risk of cancer. London: World Cancer Research Fund International; 2018.

40. Henry L. Effect of malnutrition on cancer patients. In: Nutrition Cancer. Chichester, UK: Wiley; 2011. p. 45–82.

41. Boltong A, Aranda S, Keast R, et al. A prospective cohort study of the effects of adjuvant breast cancer chemotherapy on taste function, food liking, appetite and associated nutritional outcomes. PLoS One. 2014;9(7):1–9. https://doi.org/10.1371/journal.pone.0103512.

42. Fearon K, Strasser F, Anker SD, et al. Definition and classification of cancer cachexia: an international consensus. Lancet Oncol. 2011;12(5):489–95. https://doi.org/10.1016/S1470-2045(10)70218-7.

43. Mente A, De Koning L. Shannon HS., Anand SS. B c d. a systematic review of the evidence supporting a causal link between dietary factors and coronary heart disease. Arch Intern Med. 2009;169(7):659–69. https://doi.org/10.1001/archinternmed.2009.38.

44. Rodríguez-Monforte M, Flores-Mateo G, Sánchez E. Dietary patterns and CVD: a systematic review and meta-analysis of observational studies. Br J Nutr. 2015;114(09):1341–59. https://doi.org/10.1017/S0007114515003177.

45. Estruch R, Ros E, Salas-Salvadó J, et al. Primary prevention of cardiovascular disease with a Mediterranean Diet supplemented with extra-virgin olive oil or nuts. N Engl J Med. 2018;378(25):e34. https://doi.org/10.1056/NEJMoa1800389.

46. De Lorgeril M, Salen P, Martin JL, Monjaud I, Delaye J, Mamelle N. Mediterranean diet, traditional risk factors, and the rate of cardiovascular complications after myocardial infarction: final report of the Lyon Diet Heart Study. Circulation. 1999;99(6):779–85. https://doi.org/10.1161/01.CIR.99.6.779.

47. Estruch R, Ros E, Salas-Salvadó J, et al. Primary prevention of cardiovascular disease with a Mediterranean diet. N Engl J Med. 2013;368(14):1279–90. https://doi.org/10.1056/NEJMoa1200303.

48. Buist AS, McBurnie MA, Vollmer WM, et al. International variation in the prevalence of COPD (the BOLD study): a population-based prevalence study. Lancet. 2007;370(9589):741–50. https://doi.org/10.1016/S0140-6736(07)61377-4.

49. Fukuchi Y, Nishimura M, Ichinose M, et al. COPD in Japan: the Nippon COPD epidemiology study. Respirology. 2004;9(4):458–65. https://doi.org/10.1111/j.1440-1843.2004.00637.x.

50. Zheng P, Shu L, Si C, Zhang X, Yu X, Gao W. Dietary patterns and chronic obstructive pulmonary disease: a meta-analysis. COPD J Chronic Obstr Pulm Dis. 2016;13(4):515–22.

51. Dogu B, Sirzai H, Usen A, Yilmaz F, Kuran B. Comparison of body composition, nutritional status, functional status, and quality of life between osteoporotic and osteopenic postmenopausal women. Med. 2015;51(3):173–9. https://doi.org/10.1016/j.medici.2015.05.003.

52. Tucker KL, Hannan MT, Kiel DP. The acid-base hypothesis: Diet and bone in the Framingham osteoporosis study. Eur J Nutr. 2001;40(5):231–7. https://doi.org/10.1007/s394-001-8350-8.

53. Hodges S, Akesson K, Vergnaud P, Obrant K, Delmas P. Circulating levels of vitamins K1 and K2 decreased in elderly women with hip fracture. J Bone Miner Res. 1993;8(10):1241–5.

54. Feskanich D, Weber P, Willett WC, Rockett H, Booth SL, Colditz GA. Vitamin K intake and hip fractures in women: a prospective study. Am J Clin Nutr. 1999;69(1):74–9. https://doi.org/10.1093/ajcn/69.1.74.

55. Morley JE, Vellas B, van Kan GA, et al. Frailty consensus: a call to action. J Am Med Dir Assoc.

2013;14(6):392–7. https://doi.org/10.1016/j.
jamda.2013.03.022.

56. Andela RM, Dijkstra A, Slaets JPJ, Sanderman
R. Prevalence of frailty on clinical wards: Description
and implications. Int J Nurs Pract. 2010;16(1):14–9.
https://doi.org/10.1111/j.1440-172X.2009.01807.x.

57. Kobayashi S, Asakura K, Suga H, Sasaki S. High
protein intake is associated with low prevalence of
frailty among old Japanese women: a multicenter
cross-sectional study. Nutr J. 2013;12:164.

58. Kim HK, Suzuki T, Saito K, et al. Effects of exercise
and amino acid supplementation on body composition and physical function in community-dwelling
elderly Japanese sarcopenic women: A randomized
controlled trial. J Am Geriatr Soc. 2012;60(1):16–23.
https://doi.org/10.1111/j.1532-5415.2011.03776.x.

59. Bales CW, Ritchie CS. Sarcopenia, weight loss, and
nutritional frailty in the elderly. Annu Rev Nutr.
2002;22:309–23. https://doi.org/10.1146/annurev.
nutr.22.010402.102715.

60. Paddon-Jones D, Rasmussen BB. Dietary protein
recommendations and the prevention of sarcopenia.
Curr Opin Clin Nutr Metab Care. 2009;12(1):86–90.
https://doi.org/10.1097/MCO.0b013e32831cef8b.

61. Bischoff-Ferrari H, Dawson-Hughes B, Staehelin H,
et al. Fall prevention with supplemental and active
forms of vitamin D: a meta-analysis of randomised
controlled trials. Br Med J. 2009;339:b3692.

62. Volkert D, Lochs H, Dejong C, et al. ESPEN guidelines on enteral nutrition: gastroenterology. Clin
Nutr. 2006;25(2):260–74. https://doi.org/10.1016/j.
clnu.2006.01.007.

63. Abizanda P, López MD, García VP, et al. Effects of
an oral nutritional supplementation plus physical
exercise intervention on the physical function, nutritional status, and quality of life in frail institutional-
ized older adults: the activnes study. J Am Med Dir
Assoc. 2015;16(5):439. https://doi.org/10.1016/j.
jamda.2015.02.005.

64. Morley JE, Anker SD, von Haehling S. Prevalence,
incidence, and clinical impact of sarcopenia: facts,
numbers, and epidemiology—update 2014. J
Cachexia Sarcopenia Muscle. 2014;5(4):253–9.
https://doi.org/10.1007/s13539-014-0161-y.

65. ter Borg S, de Groot LCPGM, Mijnarends DM, et al.
Differences in nutrient intake and biochemical nutrient status between sarcopenic and nonsarcopenic
older adults - results from the Maastricht Sarcopenia
Study. J Am Med Dir Assoc. 2016;17(5):393–401.
https://doi.org/10.1016/j.jamda.2015.12.015.

66. Shafiee G, Keshtkar A, Soltani A, Ahadi Z, Larijani
B, Heshmat R. Prevalence of sarcopenia in the
world: a systematic review and meta-analysis of
general population studies. J Diabetes Metab
Disord. 2017;16(1):1–10. https://doi.org/10.1186/
s40200-017-0302-x.

67. Oh C, Jeon BH, Reid Storm SN, Jho S, No JK. The
most effective factors to offset sarcopenia and obesity in the older Korean: physical activity, vitamin
D, and protein intake. Nutrition. 2017;33:169–73.
https://doi.org/10.1016/j.nut.2016.06.004.

68. Sakuma K, Yamaguchi A. Recent advances in phar-
macological, hormonal, and nutritional intervention for sarcopenia. Pflugers Arch Eur J Physiol.
2018;470(3):449–60. https://doi.org/10.1007/
s00424-017-2077-9.

69. Dillon EL, Sheffield-Moore M, Paddon-Jones D,
et al. Amino acid supplementation increases lean
body mass, basal muscle protein synthesis, and
insulin-like growth factor-I expression in older
women. J Clin Endocrinol Metab. 2009;94(5):1630–
7. https://doi.org/10.1210/jc.2008-1564.

70. Borsheim E, Bui Q, Tissier S, Kobayashi H, Ferrando
A, Wolfe R. Effect of amino acid supplementation
on muscle mass, strength and physical function in
elderly. Clin Nutr. 2009;6(2):247–53. https://doi.
org/10.1111/j.1743-6109.2008.01122.x.Endothelial.

71. Li Z, Heber D. Sarcopenic obesity in the
elderly and strategies for weight management. Nutr Rev. 2012;70(1):57–64. https://doi.
org/10.1111/j.1753-4887.2011.00453.x.

72. Sheard JM, Ash S, Silburn PA, Kerr GK. Prevalence
of malnutrition in Parkinson's disease: a systematic
review. Nutr Rev. 2011;69(9):520–32. https://doi.
org/10.1111/j.1753-4887.2011.00413.x.

73. Barichella M, Cereda E, Cassani E, et al. Dietary
habits and neurological features of Parkinson's disease patients: implications for practice. Clin Nutr.
2017;36(4):1054–61. https://doi.org/10.1016/j.
clnu.2016.06.020.

74. Seidl SE, Santiago JA, Bilyk H, Potashkin JA. The
emerging role of nutrition in Parkinson's disease.
Front Aging Neurosci. 2014;6:1–14. https://doi.
org/10.3389/fnagi.2014.00036.

75. Chen X, Maguire B, Brodaty H, O'Leary
F. Dietary patterns and cognitive health in older
adults: a systematic review. J Alzheimers Dis.
2019;67(2):583–619.

76. Prickett C, Brennan L, Stolwyk R. Examining the
relationship between obesity and cognitive function: a systematic literature review. Obes Res Clin
Pract. 2015;9(2):93–113. https://doi.org/10.1016/j.
orcp.2014.05.001.

77. Douglas JW, Lawrence JC. Environmental considerations for improving nutritional status in older adults
with dementia: a narrative review. J Acad Nutr Diet.
2015;115(11):1815–31. https://doi.org/10.1016/j.
jand.2015.06.376.

78. Nieuwenhuizen WF, Weenen H, Rigby P,
Hetherington MM. Older adults and patients in
need of nutritional support: review of current treatment options and factors influencing nutritional
intake. Clin Nutr. 2010;29(2):160–9. https://doi.
org/10.1016/j.clnu.2009.09.003.

79. Herke M, Burckhardt M, Wustmann T, Watzke
S, Fink A, Langer G. Environmental and behavioural modifications for improving food and
fluid intake in people with dementia. Cochrane
Database Syst Rev. 2015;7:CD011542. https://doi.
org/10.1002/14651858.CD011542.

80. World Health Organization, States F and AO of the
UN. Risk assessment of Listeria monocytogenes in

ready-to-eat foods. Jt FAO/WHO Expert Consult Risk Assess Microbiol Hazards Foods. 2004. p. 78-86.

81. Strausbaugh LJ. Emerging health care-associated infections in the geriatric population. Emerg Infect Dis. 2001;7(2):268–71. https://doi.org/10.3201/eid0702.700268.

82. Lund BM, O'Brien SJ. The occurrence and prevention of foodborne disease in vulnerable people. Foodborne Pathog Dis. 2011;8(9):961–73. https://doi.org/10.1089/fpd.2011.0860.

83. Lesourd BM, Mazari L. Immune responses during recovery from protein-energy malnutrition. Clin Nutr. 1997;16(SUPPL. 1):37–46. https://doi.org/10.1016/S0261-5614(97)80047-7.

84. Noble N, Paul C, Turon H, Oldmeadow C. Which modifiable health risk behaviours are related? A systematic review of the clustering of smoking, nutrition, alcohol and physical activity ('SNAP') health risk factors. Prev Med. 2015;81:16–41. https://doi.org/10.1016/j.ypmed.2015.07.003.

85. Herghelegiu AM, Moser A, Prada GI, Born S, Wilhelm M, Stuck AE. Effects of health risk assessment and counselling on physical activity in older people: a pragmatic randomised trial. PLoS One. 2017;12(7):e0181371. https://doi.org/10.1371/journal.pone.0181371.

86. Pilgrim A, Robinson S, Sayer AA, Roberts H. Europe PMC funders group: an overview of appetite decline in older people. Nurs Older People. 2015;27(5):29–35. https://doi.org/10.7748/nop.27.5.29.e697.An.

87. de Vries NM, van Ravensberg CD, Hobbelen JSM, Olde Rikkert MGM, Staal JB. Nijhuis-van der Sanden MWG. Effects of physical exercise therapy on mobility, physical functioning, physical activity and quality of life in community-dwelling older adults with impaired mobility, physical disability and/or multi-morbidity: a meta-analysis. Ageing Res Rev. 2012;11(1):136–49. https://doi.org/10.1016/j.arr.2011.11.002.

88. Forster A, Samaras N, Gold G, Samaras D. Oropharyngeal dysphagia in older adults: a review. Eur Geriatic Med. 2011;2(6):356–62.

89. Carrión S, Cabré M, Monteis R, et al. Oropharyngeal dysphagia is a prevalent risk factor for malnutrition in a cohort of older patients admitted with an acute disease to a general hospital. Clin Nutr. 2015;34(3):436–42. https://doi.org/10.1016/j.clnu.2014.04.014.

90. Mann T, Heuberger R, Wong H. The association between chewing and swallowing difficulties and nutritional status in older adults. Aust Dent J. 2013;58(2):200–6. https://doi.org/10.1111/adj.12064.

91. Matear DW, Locker D, Stephens M, Lawrence HP. Associations between xerostomia and health status indicators in the elderly. J R Soc Promot Heal. 2006;126(2):79–85. https://doi.org/10.1177/1466424006063183.

92. Fávaro-moreira NC, Krausch-hofmann S, Matthys C, et al. Risk factors for malnutrition in older adults: a systematic review of the literature based on longitudinal data. Am Soc Nutr. 2016;7(6):507–22. https://doi.org/10.3945/an.115.011254.delayed.

93. Wong CW. Vitamin B12 deficiency in the elderly: Is it worth screening? Hong Kong Med J. 2015;21(2):155–64. https://doi.org/10.12809/hkmj144383.

94. Muurinen SM, Soini HH, Suominen MH, Saarela RKT, Savikko NM, Pitkälä KH. Vision impairment and nutritional status among older assisted living residents. Arch Gerontol Geriatr. 2014;58(3):384–7. https://doi.org/10.1016/j.archger.2013.12.002.

95. Campos S, Doxey J, Hammond D. Nutrition labels on pre-packaged foods: a systematic review. Public Health Nutr. 2011;14(8):1496–506. https://doi.org/10.1017/S1368980010003290.

96. Fukanga A, Uematsu H, Sugimoto K. Influences of aging on taste perception and oral somatic sensation. J Gerontol A Biol Sci Med Sci. 2005;60(1):109–13.

97. Song X, Giacalone D, Bølling Johansen SM, Frøst MB, Bredie WLP. Changes in orosensory perception related to aging and strategies for counteracting its influence on food preferences among older adults. Trends Food Sci Technol. 2016;53:49–59. https://doi.org/10.1016/j.tifs.2016.04.004.

98. McKenna G, Burke FM. Age-related oral changes. Dent Update. 2010;37(8):519–23. https://doi.org/10.12968/denu.2010.37.8.519.

99. Malafarina V, Uriz-Otano F, Gil-Guerrero L, Iniesta R. The anorexia of ageing: physiopathology, prevalence, associated comorbidity and mortality. A systematic review. Maturitas. 2013;74(4):293–302. https://doi.org/10.1016/j.maturitas.2013.01.016.

100. MacIntosh CG, Morley JE, Wishart J, et al. Effect of exogenous cholecystokinin (CCK)-8 on food intake and plasma CCK, leptin, and insulin concentrations in older and young adults: evidence for increased CCK activity as a cause of the anorexia of aging. J Clin Endocrinol Metab. 2001;86(12):5830–7.

101. Polyakova M, Sonnabend N, Sander C, et al. Prevalence of minor depression in elderly persons with and without mild cognitive impairment: a systematic review. J Affect Disord. 2014;152-154(1):28–38. https://doi.org/10.1016/j.jad.2013.09.016.

102. Clarke DM, Currie KC. Depression, anxiety and their relationship with chronic diseases: a review of the epidemiology, risk and treatment evidence. Med J Aust. 2009;190(7 Suppl):S54–60.

103. Ahmadi SM, Mohammadi MR, Mostafavi SA, et al. Dependence of the geriatric depression on nutritional status and anthropometric indices in elderly population. Iran J Psychiatry. 2013;8(2):92–6. https://doi.org/10.1027/0200095.

104. Vafaei Z, Mokhtari H, Moeini M. Malnutrition is associated with depression in rural elderly population. J Res Med Sci. 2013;18(1):S15–9.

105. Naidoo I, Charlton KE, Esterhuizen TM, Cassim B. High risk of malnutrition associated with depres-

sive symptoms in older South Africans living in KwaZulu-Natal, South Africa: a cross-sectional survey. J Health Popul Nutr. 2015;33(1):1–8. https://doi.org/10.1186/s41043-015-0030-0.

106. Kaner G, Soylu M, Yüksel N, Inanç N, Ongan D, Başmısırlı E. Evaluation of nutritional status of patients with depression. Biomed Res Int. 2015;2015:521481. https://doi.org/10.1155/2015/521481.

107. Weber-Hamann B, Werner M, Hentschel F, et al. Metabolic changes in elderly patients with major depression: evidence for increased accumulation of visceral fat at follow-up. Psychoneuroendocrinology. 2006;31(3):347–54. https://doi.org/10.1016/j.psyneuen.2005.08.014.

108. Holt-Lunstad J, Smith TB, Baker M, Harris T, Stephenson D. Loneliness and social isolation as risk factors for mortality: a meta-analytic review. Perspect Psychol Sci. 2015;10(2):227–37. https://doi.org/10.1177/1745691614568352.

109. Locher JL, Robinson CO, Bailey FA, et al. The Contribution of Social Factors to Undereating in Older Adults with Cancer. J Support Oncol. 2009;7(5):168–73.

110. Ramic E, Pranjic N, Batic-Mujanovic O, Karic E, Alibasic E, Alic A. The effect of loneliness on malnutrition in elderly population. Med Arh. 2011;65(2):92–5.

111. Harrington J, Fitzgerald AP, Layte R, Lutomski J, Molcho M, Perry IJ. Sociodemographic, health and lifestyle predictors of poor diets. Public Health Nutr. 2011;14(12):2166–75. https://doi.org/10.1017/S136898001100098X.

112. Conklin AI, Maguire ER, Monsivais P. Economic determinants of diet in older adults: systematic review. J Epidemiol Community Health. 2013;67(9):721–7. https://doi.org/10.1136/jech-2013-202513.

113. Kobayashi LC, Wardle J, Wolf MS, Von Wagner C. Aging and functional health literacy: a systematic review and meta-analysis. J Gerontol - Ser B Psychol Sci Soc Sci. 2016;71(3):445–57. https://doi.org/10.1093/geronb/gbu161.

114. De Irala-Estévez J, Groth M, Johansson L, Oltersdorf U, Prättälä R, Martínez-González MA. A systematic review of socio-economic differences in food habits in Europe: consumption of fruit and vegetables. Eur J Clin Nutr. 2000;54(9):706–14. https://doi.org/10.1038/sj.ejcn.1601080.

Relationship Between Periodontal Disease and Nutrition

6

Lewis Winning and Ciarán Moore

Abstract

Periodontitis has been defined as "a chronic multifactorial inflammatory disease associated with dysbiotic plaque biofilms and characterized by progressive destruction of the tooth supporting apparatus". Epidemiological data suggests that periodontitis affects 45–50% of all adults, with severe periodontitis affecting 11.2% of the world's population, thus representing a significant public health challenge. In addition to well-established local and systemic risk factors for periodontal disease, attention has recently turned to the role of nutrition in disease development. The aim of this chapter is to discuss the evidence of the impact macro- and micronutrient malnutrition may have on periodontal diseases.

L. Winning (✉)
Dublin Dental University Hospital, Trinity College Dublin, The University of Dublin, Dublin, Ireland
e-mail: lewis.winning@dental.tcd.ie

C. Moore
Centre for Public Health, School of Medicine, Dentistry and Biomedical Sciences, Queen's University Belfast, Belfast, United Kingdom

6.1 Periodontal Disease

Periodontal disease is a group term used to describe a range of diseases that affect the periodontal tissues including the gingivae, alveolar bone, periodontal ligament, and root cementum. Gingivitis is the most commonly observed type of periodontal disease and refers to inflammation limited to the gingival tissues. Gingivitis is caused by dental plaque bacteria accumulating on tooth surfaces adjacent to the gingivae and is described as *reversible* in nature, as the implementation of adequate oral hygiene will cause the gum tissue to return to normal health. Most of the population are likely to exhibit clinical signs of gingivitis at some point in their lives. Periodontitis is a multifactorial inflammatory disease characterised by *irreversible* progressive destruction of the tooth-supporting structures including the periodontal attachment and alveolar bone (Figs. 6.1 and 6.2). Globally, severe periodontitis is the sixth most prevalent disease, affecting 11.2% of the population [1]. Whilst the pathogenesis of periodontitis is complex and not completely understood, there is substantial evidence that it arises as a result of an imbalance in the host inflammatory/immune response to dental plaque bacteria.

Diet has been both directly and indirectly implicated in periodontal disease for a number of years [2, 3]. It is only more recently, however, that understanding into the potential mechanisms

© Springer Nature Switzerland AG 2021
G. McKenna (ed.), *Nutrition and Oral Health*, https://doi.org/10.1007/978-3-030-80526-5_6

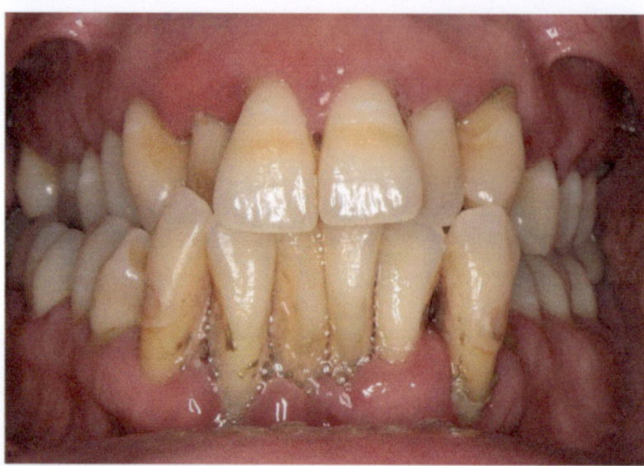

Fig. 6.1 Clinical appearance of a patient with generalized periodontitis

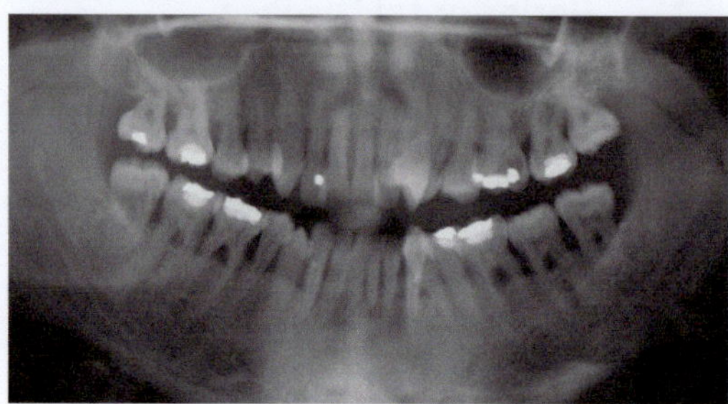

Fig. 6.2 Radiographic appearance of a patient with generalized periodontitis displaying associated loss of alveolar bone

by which it can modulate the host's immune/inflammatory systems and affect periodontal inflammation has been advanced. Nutrients derived from the diet perform as antioxidants, coenzymes in energy production and metabolic processes, and components of tissue structures that help to maintain normal body homeostatic processes including periodontal functions. Depletion or lack of availability of nutrients can give rise to malnutrition at either the macro- or the micronutrient level. Both are detrimental to periodontal health as well as to general health [4, 5]. With this growing body of evidence, the 2011 European Workshop on Periodontology went as far as suggesting dietary recommendations for the prevention and treatment of periodontal disease. These included increasing dietary fibre, fish oil, fruits, and vegetables and reducing intake of refined sugars [6].

6.2 Macronutrient Malnutrition and Periodontal Disease

6.2.1 Carbohydrates

Carbohydrates, including glucose, are needed for adequate cellular functioning and for normal physiological processes such as the construction of the periodontal tissues [7]. The excessive intake of carbohydrate, i.e. a diet consisting of 30–50% or more of carbohydrate, however, may be associated with the development of periodontal disease [8]. Increased consumption of refined sugars can inhibit tissue repair and promote oxidative stress, microbial dysbiosis, chronic inflammation, and cellular apoptosis [9–14]. Several studies have demonstrated an increase in gingival bleeding associated with the increased consumption of carbohydrates [15, 16]. Furthermore, the adoption of a carbohydrate-restricted diet has been shown to decrease levels of gingival and periodontal inflammation among humans, as well as slow rates of alveolar bone loss in animals [17, 18]. Diabetes mellitus and obesity, both of which may be related to the excessive dietary intake of carbohydrate, are also associated with an increased risk of developing periodontitis [19, 20]. In contrast, increased frequency of intake of dietary fibre (plant-derived cellulose, polysaccharides, and lignins that cannot be completely digested by humans) has been associated with a lower odds of gingival bleeding in adolescent girls [21, 22].

6.2.2 Protein

Proteins such as collagen form a major component of periodontal connective tissue, dental hard tissue, and alveolar bone [21]. They are also needed for the effective function of the humoral and cell-mediated immune systems, as well as complement and other host defence mechanisms [7]. Numerous studies have shown protein deprivation to be associated with the degeneration of gingival and periodontal connective tissue, osteoporosis of alveolar bone, retardation in cemental deposition, and consequently periodontitis and tooth loss [23, 24].

6.2.3   Fats

Omega-3 fatty acids are a key constituent of host cell membranes and are essential for the maintenance of membrane integrity. These long-chain polyunsaturated fatty acids are also required for the modulation of immune function and have been demonstrated to have anti-inflammatory properties [25]. Increased intake of omega-3 through the consumption of fish oil, sea fish, or flaxseed oil has been associated with a reduction in the risk of periodontitis [26–28]. Moreover, randomised controlled trials conducted by Deore et al. and El-Sharkawy et al. both demonstrated a greater reduction in periodontal probing pocket depths and increased clinical attachment gain for patients treated by non-surgical periodontal treatment and supplementary omega-3, compared to patients treated by non-surgical periodontal treatment alone [29, 30].

In contrast to omega-3, the increased consumption of omega-6 fatty acids (predominantly sourced from vegetable oils) has been associated with poorer periodontal outcomes. Increased dietary intake of saturated fats has also been found to be directly correlated with an increased incidence of periodontitis. Saturated fats may increase the severity of inflammation within the periodontium and may accelerate the resorption of alveolar bone [31]. Moreover, elevated levels of blood lipid have also been associated with an increased risk of periodontitis [32].

In an observational study conducted by Hamasaki et al., the total percentage intake of calories from fat was found to be an important nutrient factor associated with the risk of periodontitis. They discovered that patients with advanced periodontitis tended to have a diet consisting of a greater percentage intake of carbohydrate and a lower percentage intake of total fat [26].

6.3   Micronutrient Malnutrition and Periodontal Disease

6.3.1   Vitamin A/Carotenoids

(*Including preformed retinoids, proretinoid carotenoids (e.g. α-carotene, β-carotene, and β-cryptoxanthin) and non-proretinoid carotenoids (e.g. lutein, lycopene, zeaxanthin, astaxanthin, and canthaxanthin)*)

Vitamin A is essential for epithelial cell proliferation, prevention of infection, and adequate immune function [21]. Additionally, carotenoids have been demonstrated to possess anti-inflammatory properties [33]. Deficiency of vitamin A is rare in developed countries; however, it is much more prevalent in developing countries. In 1963, Russell determined that populations with a high prevalence of periodontitis were typically deficient in vitamin A [34]. A similar study by Waerhaug, however, found no association between vitamin A deficiency and periodontitis [35]. In the Third United States National Health and Nutrition Examination Survey, a weak inverse association between the intake of proretinoid carotenoids (α-carotene, β-carotene, and β-cryptoxanthin) and mild periodontitis was determined [36]. Total antioxidant capacity, to which serum vitamin A concentration was a contributor, was associated with a lower odds of developing severe periodontitis; however, no association was found between periodontitis and serum vitamin A concentration alone. Linden et al. found low levels of carotenoids to be associated with a significantly increased risk of moderate periodontitis, and low levels of β-carotene and β-cryptoxanthin to be associated with an increased risk of generalised severe periodontitis [37]. Increased dietary consumption of β-carotene, or the administration of lycopene (either locally or systemically), in addition to non-surgical periodontal treatment, has been shown to be associated with an improved response to treatment [38]. Currently, there exists a paucity of studies regarding vitamin A supplementation and the response to periodontal therapy, presumably, as a result of the risk of liver toxicity associated with excessive serum levels of vitamin A.

6.3.2 Vitamin B Complex

(Including thiamine (B1), riboflavin (B2), niacin (B3), pantothenic acid (B5), pyridoxine (B6), biotin (B7), folic acid (B9 or Bc), and cobalamin (B12))

B complex vitamins are needed for adequate host metabolism, muscle development, construction of red blood cells, and synthesis of collagen. Low serum levels of vitamin B12 have been associated with greater levels of clinical attachment loss, and an increased risk of tooth loss, among patients [39]. Low serum folate levels have also been demonstrated to be associated with the development of periodontitis in older adults [40]. Periodontitis patients who smoke have been shown to have lower serum folate levels than both periodontitis patients who are non-smokers and periodontally healthy patients [41]. In a study by Neiva et al., vitamin B complex supplementation was associated with improved clinical attachment levels following periodontal surgery in patients with periodontitis [42]. Furthermore, the local or systemic delivery of folate has also been shown to reduce gingival inflammation among patients with plaque-induced gingivitis, pregnancy gingivitis, and periodontitis [43].

6.3.3 Vitamin C (Ascorbic Acid)

Vitamin C is considered an effective antioxidant and is essential for collagen synthesis and regulation of inflammation. Scurvy, a vitamin C deficiency disease characterised by gingival bleeding and tooth mobility secondary to impaired collagen and connective tissue synthesis, was widely prevalent in the eighteenth century. Its prevalence now is much rarer, particularly in developed countries. In developing countries, deficiency of serum vitamin C has been shown to be associated with increased clinical attachment

loss [44]. Moreover, serum vitamin C levels have also been shown to be inversely associated with periodontitis, particularly among patients who have never smoked [45]. The habit of smoking has also been associated with decreased serum vitamin C levels in patients with periodontitis, compared to non-smoking periodontitis patients and non-smoking periodontally healthy patients [46]. Increased intake of vitamin C from dietary sources, or supplementation, has been shown to increase serum vitamin C levels in non-smokers, and to reduce gingival bleeding in patients with gingivitis, periodontitis, and diabetes mellitus [47, 48].

6.3.4 Vitamin D

Vitamin D is important for the absorption of dietary calcium, bone metabolism, and appropriate modulation of the host innate and adaptive immune and inflammatory responses. Based on data from the Third United States National Health and Nutrition Examination Survey, researchers discovered that patients with high serum levels of vitamin D had less alveolar bone loss (when over the age of 50 years), reduced bleeding on probing, and decreased clinical attachment loss and fewer missing teeth (among postmenopausal women on hormone replacement therapy), in comparison to patients with low serum levels of vitamin D [49, 50]. Other studies have demonstrated that periodontitis patients may have lower blood levels of vitamin D compared to periodontally healthy patients [51–53]. Indeed, a study by Zhan et al. showed an inverse correlation between a patient's serum vitamin D level and the risk of tooth loss [53].

6.3.5 Vitamin E

Vitamin E is an important antioxidant and possesses anti-inflammatory and anti-thrombotic properties. In a study by Chapple et al., no association was found between the prevalence of periodontitis and serum vitamin E levels, using data obtained from the Third United States National

Health and Nutrition Examination Survey [36]. In contrast, Zong et al. demonstrated a non-linear inverse relationship between serum alpha-tocopherol levels and severity of periodontitis among patients with low serum vitamin E levels [54]. Increased dietary intake or supplementation with vitamin E has been shown to reduce periodontal disease progression, decrease periodontal inflammation, and improve the response to periodontal treatment, among periodontitis patients [5, 38, 55, 56].

6.3.6 Calcium

Calcium, in the form of hydroxyapatite, is the primary constituent of bone and dental hard tissue [5]. Intracellular levels of calcium are also important for the regulation of membrane permeability, muscle contraction, and DNA synthesis [5, 21]. Sources of absorbable calcium in the diet include dairy products, as well as broccoli, kale, almonds, dried apricots, and mineral water [57]. Smoking has also been shown to reduce calcium absorption [58]. Low dietary intake of calcium has been associated with an increased severity of periodontitis, higher rates of alveolar bone loss, and increased tooth loss among patients [59–61]. Furthermore, an inverse relationship between the intake of dairy products and the prevalence and severity of periodontitis has also been determined [59, 62]. Al-Zahrani et al. demonstrated that patients with a high dietary intake of dairy products were 20% less likely to have periodontitis than patients with a low dietary intake of dairy products [62]. Other studies that have explored the relationship between periodontitis and intake of calcium and/or dairy products, however, have proved inconclusive [63, 64]. Serum calcium levels have been demonstrated to be inversely associated with the progression of periodontitis [65]. Moreover, calcium supplementation has been shown to reduce the risk of tooth loss, and is also associated with an improved response to non-surgical periodontal therapy when given in combination with supplementary vitamin D [60, 66–68].

6.3.7 Magnesium

Magnesium is needed for cell metabolism, regulation of intracellular calcium levels, vitamin metabolism, hormone and DNA synthesis, and bone mineralisation [5]. Meisel et al. demonstrated that nutritional magnesium supplementation may be associated with decreased clinical attachment loss and reduced tooth loss [69]. Pushparani et al. found that diabetic patients with or without periodontitis, and non-diabetic patients with periodontitis, had lower serum magnesium levels compared to healthy control patients [70]. Shetty et al. demonstrated similar findings, as well as a significant increase in serum magnesium among diabetic patients with or without periodontitis, and non-diabetic patients with periodontitis, 3 weeks after non-surgical periodontal treatment [71]. An increased serum magnesium/calcium ratio, however, has been associated with an increased risk of periodontitis progression [69, 72].

6.3.8 Iron

Iron is essential for the formation of haemoglobin and oxygen transport around the body. Periodontitis patients have been demonstrated to have a lower number of red blood cells and lower haemoglobin than healthy patients [73]. The progression of periodontitis may also be associated with a decrease in red cell count [74]. It has been speculated that the chronic inflammatory state of periodontitis may stimulate the suppression of erythropoiesis [5, 75]. Moreover, the treatment of periodontitis has been shown to improve haematological parameters [75, 76]. Periodontitis patients with iron-deficiency anaemia have been demonstrated to have a higher number of bleeding sites, greater probing pocket depths, and increased clinical attachment loss, compared to non-anaemic periodontitis patients [77]. Low iron intake and low serum iron have also been associated with periodontitis in women and periodontitis in diabetic patients, respectively [45, 78]. These findings were not replicated, however, by Gautam et al. and Enhos et al. [79, 80].

6.4 Alcohol

Several studies have suggested that moderate or heavy alcohol consumption increases the risk of clinical attachment loss [81–83]. Jansson, and Kongstad et al., however, reported contradictory findings [84, 85]. Presently, it remains unclear how alcohol intake affects periodontal disease risk [21].

6.5 Conclusions

It must be acknowledged that there are significant limitations in relation to many of the studies discussed in this chapter. In numerous studies, dietary intake was assessed using self-reported questionnaires, raising issues around data reliability. Furthermore, in many instances, subgroups of patients (e.g. pregnant or diabetic patients) were analysed, limiting the generalisability of each study's findings.

Concerns persist regarding the strength of the current available evidence and whether it is sufficient to support a therapeutic role for diet and nutrition in periodontal disease management [5, 21]. More research is obviously needed in this area. Nevertheless, dental professionals can play an important holistic role in patient care by assessing the nutritional needs of their patients, particularly as they tend to see their patients on a regular recall basis, and are advised to provide dietary advice in line with the "Eatwell Guide", the recommendations of the Seventh European Workshop on Periodontology, and Public Health England's "Delivering Better Oral Health: An Evidence-Based Toolkit for Prevention" [86–89].

References

1. Kassebaum NJ, Bernabé E, Dahiya M, Bhandari B, Murray CJL, Marcenes W. Global burden of severe periodontitis in 1990-2010. J Dent Res. 2014;93(11):1045–53. https://doi.org/10.1177/0022034514552491.

2. Enwonwu CO. Interface of malnutrition and periodontal diseases. Am J Clin Nutr. 1995;61(2):430S–6S. https://doi.org/10.1093/ajcn/61.2.430s.

3. Wright DM, McKenna G, Nugent A, Winning L, Linden GJ, Woodside JV. Association between diet and periodontitis: a cross-sectional study of 10,000 NHANES participants. Am J Clin Nutr. 2020;112(6):1485–91. https://doi.org/10.1093/ajcn/nqaa266.

4. Enwonwu CO, Phillips RS, Falkler WA. Nutrition and oral infectious diseases: state of the science. Compend Contin Educ Dent. 2002;23(5):431–4.

5. Dommisch H, Kuzmanova D, Jönsson D, Grant M, Chapple I. Effect of micronutrient malnutrition on periodontal disease and periodontal therapy. Periodontol 2000. 2018;78(1):129–53. https://doi.org/10.1111/prd.12233.

6. Tonetti MS, Chapple ILC. Biological approaches to the development of novel periodontal therapies - Consensus of the Seventh European Workshop on Periodontology. J Clin Periodontol. 2011;38:114–8. https://doi.org/10.1111/j.1600-051X.2010.01675.x.

7. Schifferle RE. Periodontal disease and nutrition: Separating the evidence from current fads. Periodontol 2000. 2009;50(1):78–89. https://doi.org/10.1111/j.1600-0757.2008.00297.x.

8. Hujoel P. Dietary carbohydrates and dental-systemic diseases. J Dent Res. 2009;88(6):490–502. https://doi.org/10.1177/0022034509337700.

9. Chapple ILC. Potential mechanisms underpinning the nutritional modulation of periodontal inflammation. J Am Dent Assoc. 2009;140(2):178–84. https://doi.org/10.14219/jada.archive.2009.0131.

10. Liu J, Jiang Y, Mao J, Gu B, Liu H, Fang B. High levels of glucose induces a dose-dependent apoptosis in human periodontal ligament fibroblasts by activating caspase-3 signaling pathway. Appl Biochem Biotechnol. 2013;170(6):1458–71. https://doi.org/10.1007/s12010-013-0287-y.

11. Kim HS, Park JW, Yeo SI, Choi BJ, Suh JY. Effects of high glucose on cellular activity of periodontal ligament cells in vitro. Diabetes Res Clin Pract. 2006;74(1):41–7. https://doi.org/10.1016/j.diabres.2006.03.034.

12. Adler CJ, Dobney K, Weyrich LS, et al. Sequencing ancient calcified dental plaque shows changes in oral microbiota with dietary shifts of the Neolithic and Industrial revolutions. Nat Genet. 2013;45:450–5. https://doi.org/10.1038/ng.2536.

13. Bosma-Den Boer MM, Van Wetten ML, Pruimboom L. Chronic inflammatory diseases are stimulated by current lifestyle: How diet, stress levels and medication prevent our body from recovering. Nutr Metab. 2012;9(1):32. https://doi.org/10.1186/1743-7075-9-32.

14. Raindi D. Nutrition and periodontal disease. Dent Update. 2016;43(1):66–8. https://doi.org/10.12968/denu.2016.43.1.66.

15. Sidi AD, Ashley FP. Influence of frequent sugar intakes on experimental gingivitis. J Periodontol.

1984;55(7):419–23.   https://doi.org/10.1902/jop.1984.55.7.419.

16. Gaengler P, Pfister W, Sproessig M, Mirgorod M. The effects of carbohydrate-reduced diet on development of gingivitis. Clin Prev Dent. 1986;8(6):17–23.

17. Baumgartner S, Imfeld T, Schicht O, Rath C, Persson RE, Persson GR. The impact of the stone age diet on gingival conditions in the absence of oral hygiene. J Periodontol. 2009;80(5):759–68. https://doi.org/10.1902/jop.2009.080376.

18. Woelber JP, Bremer K, Vach K, et al. An oral health optimized diet can reduce gingival and periodontal inflammation in humans - a randomized controlled pilot study. BMC Oral Health. 2016;17(1):28. https://doi.org/10.1186/s12903-016-0257-1.

19. Nascimento GG, Leite FRM, Vestergaard P, Scheutz F, López R. Does diabetes increase the risk of periodontitis? A systematic review and meta-regression analysis of longitudinal prospective studies. Acta Diabetol. 2018;55(7):653–67. https://doi.org/10.1007/s00592-018-1120-4.

20. Chaffee BW, Weston SJ. Association between chronic periodontal disease and obesity: a systematic review and meta-analysis. J Periodontol. 2010;81(12):1708–24. https://doi.org/10.1902/jop.2010.100321.

21. Kaye EK. Nutrition, dietary guidelines and optimal periodontal health. Periodontol 2000. 2012;58(1):93–111. https://doi.org/10.1111/j.1600-0757.2011.00418.x.

22. Petti S, Cairella G, Tarsitani G. Nutritional variables related to gingival health in adolescent girls. Community Dent Oral Epidemiol. 2000;28(6):407–13. https://doi.org/10.1034/j.1600-0528.2000.028006407.x.

23. Pindborg JJ, Bhat M, Roed-Petersen B. Oral changes in South Indian children with severe protein deficiency with special reference to periodontal conditions. J Periodontol. 1967;38(3):218–21. https://doi.org/10.1902/jop.1967.38.3.218.

24. Hujoel PP, Lingström P. Nutrition, dental caries and periodontal disease: a narrative review. J Clin Periodontol. 2017;44:S79–84. https://doi.org/10.1111/jcpe.12672.

25. Zhao G, Etherton TD, Martin KR, Gillies PJ, West SG, Kris-Etherton PM. Dietary α-linolenic acid inhibits proinflammatory cytokine production by peripheral blood mononuclear cells in hypercholesterolemic subjects. Am J Clin Nutr. 2007;85(2):385–91. https://doi.org/10.1093/ajcn/85.2.385.

26. Hamasaki T, Kitamura M, Kawashita Y, Ando Y, Saito T. Periodontal disease and percentage of calories from fat using national data. J Periodontal Res. 2017;52(1):114–21. https://doi.org/10.1111/jre.12375.

27. Naqvi AZ, Buettner C, Phillips RS, Davis RB, Mukamal KJ. N-3 fatty acids and periodontitis in US adults. J Am Diet Assoc. 2010;110(11):1669–75. https://doi.org/10.1016/j.jada.2010.08.009.

28. Iwasaki M, Yoshihara A, Moynihan P, Watanabe R, Taylor GW, Miyazaki H. Longitudinal relationship between dietary ω-3 fatty acids and periodontal disease. Nutrition. 2010;26(11-12):1105–9. https://doi.org/10.1016/j.nut.2009.09.010.

29. Deore GD, Gurav AN, Patil R, Shete AR, Naik Tari RS, Inamdar SP. Omega 3 fatty acids as a host modulator in chronic periodontitis patients: A randomised, double-blind, placebo-controlled, clinical trial. J Periodontal Implant Sci. 2014;44(1):25–32. https://doi.org/10.5051/jpis.2014.44.1.25.

30. El-Sharkawy H, Aboelsaad N, Eliwa M, et al. Adjunctive treatment of chronic periodontitis with daily dietary supplementation with omega-3 fatty acids and low-dose aspirin. J Periodontol. 2010;81(11):1635–43. https://doi.org/10.1902/jop.2010.090628.

31. Iwasaki M, Manz MC, Moynihan P, et al. Relationship between saturated fatty acids and periodontal disease. J Dent Res. 2011;90(7):861–7. https://doi.org/10.1177/0022034511405384.

32. Lee JB, Yi HY, Bae KH. The association between periodontitis and dyslipidemia based on the fourth Korea National Health and Nutrition Examination Survey. J Clin Periodontol. 2013;40(5):437–42. https://doi.org/10.1111/jcpe.12095.

33. Raverdeau M, Mills KHG. Modulation of T cell and innate immune responses by retinoic acid. J Immunol. 2014;192(7):2953–8. https://doi.org/10.4049/jimmunol.1303245.

34. Russell AL. International nutrition surveys: a summary of preliminary dental findings. J Dent Res. 1963;42(1):233–44. https://doi.org/10.1177/00220345630420012401.

35. Waerhaug J. Prevalence of periodontal disease IR Ceylon: association with age, sex, oral hygiene, socio-economic factors, vitamin deficiencies, malnutrition, betel and tobacco consumption and ethnic group final report. Acta Odontol Scand. 1967;25(2):205–31. https://doi.org/10.3109/00016356709028749.

36. Chapple ILC, Milward MR, Dietrich T. The prevalence of inflammatory periodontitis is negatively associated with serum antioxidant concentrations. J Nutr. 2007;137(3):657–64. https://doi.org/10.1093/jn/137.3.657.

37. Linden GJ, McClean KM, Woodside JV, et al. Antioxidants and periodontitis in 60-70-year-old men. J Clin Periodontol. 2009;36(10):843–9. https://doi.org/10.1111/j.1600-051X.2009.01468.x.

38. Dodington DW, Fritz PC, Sullivan PJ, Ward WE. Higher intakes of fruits and vegetables, β-carotene, vitamin C, α-tocopherol, EPA, and DHA are positively associated with periodontal healing after nonsurgical periodontal therapy in nonsmokers but not in smokers. J Nutr. 2015;145(11):2512–9. https://doi.org/10.3945/jn.115.211524.

39. Zong G, Holtfreter B, Scott AE, et al. Serum vitamin B12 is inversely associated with periodontal progression and risk of tooth loss: a prospective cohort study. J Clin Periodontol. 2016;43(1):2–9. https://doi.org/10.1111/jcpe.12483.

40. Yu YH, Kuo HK, Lai YL. The association between serum folate levels and periodontal disease in older adults: data from the National Health and Nutrition Examination Survey 2001/02. J Am Geriatr Soc. 2007;55(1):108–13. https://doi.org/10.1111/j.1532-5415.2006.01020.x.
41. Erdemir EO, Bergstrom J. Relationship between smoking and folic acid, vitamin B12 and some haematological variables in patients with chronic periodontal disease. J Clin Periodontol. 2006;33(12):878–84. https://doi.org/10.1111/j.1600-051X.2006.01003.x.
42. Neiva RF, Steigenga J, Al-Shammari KF, Wang HL. Effects of specific nutrients on periodontal disease onset, progression and treatment. J Clin Periodontol. 2003;30(7):579–89. https://doi.org/10.1034/j.1600-051X.2003.00354.x.
43. Pack ARC, Thomson ME. Effects of topical and systemic folic acid supplementation on gingivitis in pregnancy. J Clin Periodontol. 1980;7(5):402–14. https://doi.org/10.1111/j.1600-051X.1980.tb02013.x.
44. Amaliya, Timmerman MF, Abbas F, et al. Java project on periodontal diseases: the relationship between vitamin C and the severity of periodontitis. J Clin Periodontol. 2007;34(4):299–304. https://doi.org/10.1111/j.1600-051X.2007.01053.x.
45. Park JA, Lee JH, Lee HJ, Jin BH, Bae KH. Association of Some Vitamins and Minerals with Periodontitis in a Nationally Representative Sample of Korean Young Adults. Biol Trace Elem Res. 2017;178(2):171–9. https://doi.org/10.1007/s12011-016-0914-x.
46. Staudte H, Sigusch BW, Glockmann E. Grapefruit consumption improves vitamin C status in periodontitis patients. Br Dent J. 2005;199(4):213–7. https://doi.org/10.1038/sj.bdj.4812613.
47. Gokhale NH, Acharya AB, Patil VS, Trivedi DJ, Thakur SL. A short-term evaluation of the relationship between plasma ascorbic acid levels and periodontal disease in systemically healthy and type 2 diabetes mellitus subjects. J Diet Suppl. 2013;10(2):93–104. https://doi.org/10.3109/19390211.2013.790332.
48. Leggott PJ, Robertson PB, Jacob RA, Zambon JJ, Walsh M, Armitage GC. Effects of ascorbic acid depletion and supplementation on periodontal health and subgingival microflora in humans. J Dent Res. 1991;70(12):1531–6. https://doi.org/10.1177/00220345910700121101.
49. Dietrich T, Nunn M, Dawson-Hughes B, Bischoff-Ferrari HA. Association between serum concentrations of 25-hydroxyvitamin D and gingival inflammation. Am J Clin Nutr. 2005;82(3):575–80.
50. Jonsson D, Aggarwal P, Nilsson B-O, Demmer RT. beneficial effects of hormone replacement therapy on periodontitis are vitamin D associated. J Periodontol. 1970;84(8):1048–57.
51. Antonoglou GN, Knuuttila M, Niemelä O, Raunio T, Karttunen R, Vainio O, Hedberg P, Ylöstalo P, Tervonen T. Low serum level of 1,25(OH) D is associated with chronic periodontitis. J Periodontal Res. 2015;50(2):274–80.
52. Laky M, Bertl K, Haririan H, Andrukhov O, Seemann R, Volf I, Assinger A, Gruber R, Moritz A, Rausch-Fan X. Serum levels of 25-hydroxyvitamin D are associated with periodontal disease. Clin Oral Investig. 2017;21(5):1553–8.
53. Zhan Y, Samietz S, Holtfreter B, Hannemann A, Meisel P, Nauck M, Völzke H, Wallaschofski H, Dietrich T, Kocher T. Prospective study of serum 25-hydroxy vitamin D and tooth loss. J Dent Res. 2014;93(7):639–44.
54. Zong G, Scott AE, Griffiths HR, Zock PL, Dietrich T, Newson RS. Serum α-tocopherol has a nonlinear inverse association with periodontitis among US adults. J Nutr. 2015;145(5):893–9. https://doi.org/10.3945/jn.114.203703.
55. Iwasaki M, Manz MC, Taylor GW, Yoshihara A, Miyazaki H. Relations of serum ascorbic acid and α-tocopherol to periodontal disease. J Dent Res. 2012;91(2):167–72. https://doi.org/10.1177/0022034511431702.
56. Singh N, Chander Narula S, Kumar Sharma R, Tewari S, Kumar SP. Vitamin E supplementation, superoxide dismutase status, and outcome of scaling and root planing in patients with chronic periodontitis: a randomized clinical trial. J Periodontol. 2014;85(2):242–9. https://doi.org/10.1902/jop.2013.120727.
57. European Food Safety Authority. Scientific opinion on dietary reference values for vitamin a. EFSA J. 2015;13(3):4028. https://doi.org/10.2903/j.efsa.2015.4028.
58. Rapuri PB, Gallagher JC, Balhorn KE, Ryschon KL. Smoking and bone metabolism in elderly women. Bone. 2000;27(3):429–36.
59. Adegboye AR, Christensen LB, Holm-Pedersen P, Avlund K, Boucher BJ, Heitmann BL. Intakes of calcium, vitamin D, and dairy servings and dental plaque in older Danish adults. Nutr J. 2013;12:61. https://doi.org/10.1186/1475-2891-12-61.
60. Krall EA, Wehler C, Garcia RI, Harris SS, Dawson-Hughes B. Calcium and vitamin D supplements reduce tooth loss in the elderly. Am J Med. 2001;111(6):452–6.
61. Nishida M, Grossi SG, Dunford RG, Ho AW, Trevisan M, Genco RJ. Dietary vitamin C and the risk for periodontal disease. J Periodontol. 2000;71(8):1215–23. https://doi.org/10.1902/jop.2000.71.8.1215.
62. Al-Zahrani MS. Increased intake of dairy products is related to lower periodontitis prevalence. J Periodontol. 2006;77(2):289–94. https://doi.org/10.1902/jop.2006.050082.
63. Uhrbom E, Jacobson L. Calcium and periodontitis: clinical effect of calcium medication. J Clin Periodontol. 1984;11(4):230–41.
64. Shimazaki Y, Shirota T, Uchida K, et al. Intake of dairy products and periodontal disease: the Hisayama study. J Periodontol. 2008;79(1):131–7. https://doi.org/10.1902/jop.2008.070202.
65. Amarasena N, Yoshihara A, Hirotomi T, Takano N, Miyazaki H. Association between serum calcium and

periodontal disease progression in non-institution-alized elderly. Gerodontology. 2008;25(4):245–50. https://doi.org/10.1111/j.1741-2358.2007.00211.x.

66. Krall EA, Garcia RI, Dawson-Hughes B. Increased risk of tooth loss is related to bone loss at the whole body, hip, and spine. Calcif Tissue Int. 1996;59(6):433–7.

67. Miley DD, Garcia MN, Hildebolt CF, et al. Cross-sectional study of vitamin D and calcium supplementation effects on chronic periodontitis. J Periodontol. 2009;80(9):1433–9. https://doi.org/10.1902/jop.2009.090077.

68. Garcia MN, Hildebolt CF, Miley DD, et al. One-year effects of vitamin D and calcium supplementation on chronic periodontitis. J Periodontol. 2011;82(1):25–32. https://doi.org/10.1902/jop.2010.100207.

69. Meisel P, Schwahn C, Luedemann J, John U, Kroemer HK, Kocher T. Magnesium deficiency is associated with periodontal disease. J Dent Res. 2005;84(10):937–41. https://doi.org/10.1177/154405910508401012.

70. Pushparani D, Anandan SN, Theagarayan P. Serum zinc and magnesium concentrations in type 2 diabetes mellitus with periodontitis. J Indian Soc Periodontol. 2014;18(2):187. https://doi.org/10.4103/0972-124X.131322.

71. Shetty A, Bhandary R, Thomas B, Ramesh A. A comparative evaluation of serum magnesium in diabetes mellitus type 2 patients with and without periodontitis - a clinico-biochemical study. J Clin Diagn Res. 2016;10(12):ZC59–61. https://doi.org/10.7860/JCDR/2016/21063.9078.

72. Yoshihara A, Iwasaki M, Miyazaki H. Mineral content of calcium and magnesium in the serum and longitudinal periodontal progression in Japanese elderly smokers. J Clin Periodontol. 2011;38(11):992–7. https://doi.org/10.1111/j.1600-051X.2011.01769.x.

73. Gokhale SR, Sumanth S, Padhye AM. Evaluation of blood parameters in patients with chronic periodontitis for signs of anemia. J Periodontol. 2010;81(8):1202–6. https://doi.org/10.1902/jop.2010.100079.

74. Yamamoto T, Tsuneishi M, Furuta M, Ekuni D, Morita M, Hirata Y. Relationship between decrease of erythrocyte count and progression of periodontal disease in a rural Japanese population. J Periodontol. 2011;82(1):106–13. https://doi.org/10.1902/jop.2010.100211.

75. Pradeep AR, Anuj S. Anemia of chronic disease and chronic periodontitis: does periodontal therapy have an effect on anemic status? J Periodontol. 2011;82(3):388–94. https://doi.org/10.1902/jop.2010.100336.

76. Patel M, Shakir Q, Shetty A. Interrelationship between chronic periodontitis and anemia: a 6-month follow-up study. J Indian Soc Periodontol. 2014;18(1):19. https://doi.org/10.4103/0972-124X.128194.

77. Chakraborty S, Tewari S, Sharma RK, Narula SC, Ghalaut PS, Ghalaut V. Impact of iron deficiency anemia on chronic periodontitis and superoxide dismutase activity: a cross-sectional study. J Periodontal Implant Sci. 2014;44(2):57. https://doi.org/10.5051/jpis.2014.44.2.57.

78. Pushparani DS, Nirmala S. High level of serum calcium and iron influences the risk of type 2 diabetes mellitus with periodontitis. J Asian Sci Res. 2014;4(2):70–82.

79. Gautam A, Prasad BR, Kumari S, Thomas B. Evaluation of micronutrient (zinc, copper and iron) levels in periodontitis patients with and without diabetes mellitus type 2: a biochemical study. Indian J Dent Res. 2013;24(4):468. https://doi.org/10.4103/0970-9290.118400.

80. Enhos S, Duran I, Erdem S, Buyukbas S. Relationship between iron-deficiency anemia and periodontal status in female patients. J Periodontol. 2009;80(11):1750–5. https://doi.org/10.1902/jop.2009.090209.

81. Pitiphat W, Merchant AT, Rimm EB, Joshipura KJ. Alcohol consumption increases periodontitis risk. J Dent Res. 2003;82(7):509–13. https://doi.org/10.1177/154405910308200704.

82. Tezal M, Grossi SG, Ho AW, Genco RJ. The effect of alcohol consumption on periodontal disease. J Periodontol. 2001;72(2):183–9. https://doi.org/10.1902/jop.2001.72.2.183.

83. Tezal M, Grossi SG, Ho AW, Genco RJ. Alcohol consumption and periodontal disease. The third National Health and Nutrition Examination Survey. J Clin Periodontol. 2004;31(7):484–8. https://doi.org/10.1111/j.1600-051X.2004.00503.x.

84. Jansson L. Association between alcohol consumption and dental health. J Clin Periodontol. 2008;35(5):379–84. https://doi.org/10.1111/j.1600-051X.2008.01210.x.

85. Kongstad J, Hvidtfeldt UA, Grønbaek M, Jontell M, Stoltze K, Holmstrup P. Amount and type of alcohol and periodontitis in the Copenhagen City Heart Study. J Clin Periodontol. 2008;35(12):1032–9. https://doi.org/10.1111/j.1600-051X.2008.01325.x.

86. Sanz M, Lang NP, Kinane DF, Berglundh T, Chapple I, Tonetti MS. Seventh European Workshop on Periodontology of the European Academy of Periodontology at the Parador at La Granja, Segovia, Spain. J Clin Periodontol. 2011;38:1–2. https://doi.org/10.1111/j.1600-051X.2010.01692.x.

87. British Dental Journal. Eat well, keep gums healthy, live longer. BDJ Team. 2019;6:19040.

88. Public Health England. The Eatwell Guide - A revised healthy eating model - British Nutrition Foundation. London: British Nutrition Foundation. 2016.

89. Public Health England. Delivering better oral health: an evidence-based toolkit for prevention - GOV.UK. 2017.

Impacts of Oral Rehabilitation on Nutritional Status

7

Martina Hayes, Cristiane da Mata, Francis Burke, and Gerry McKenna

Abstract

The functions of natural teeth are to enable mastication whilst also helping to form speech and provide aesthetics. Whilst the aesthetic role of teeth is becoming more important and financially rewarding for clinicians, the role of teeth in mastication is much more fundamental. Historically, incisors were developed for incising foods into a manageable bolus and molars developed to comminute the bolus to facilitate ingestion. Unfortunately, teeth can be lost, mainly due to caries, periodontal disease or trauma during a patient's lifetime whilst others are congenitally missing. This chapter examines the consequences of natural tooth loss on oral function, including mastication, and nutritional choices. It also describes the impact of replacing missing teeth with various prosthodontic treatments on mastication and nutritional status.

M. Hayes (✉) · C. da Mata · F. Burke
Cork University Dental School and Hospital,
University College Cork,
Cork, Ireland
e-mail: martina.hayes@ucc.ie

G. McKenna
Centre for Public Health, School of Medicine,
Dentistry and Biomedical Sciences, Queen's
University Belfast, Belfast, United Kingdom

7.1 Functional Consequences of Tooth Loss

7.1.1 Mastication

As natural teeth are lost, this can significantly impact patients' oral function. Research has shown that a decreased number of natural teeth results in reduced chewing ability with edentulous patients possessing lower chewing ability compared to dentate patients [1]. With a decreased number of teeth, a reduction in chewing ability can result in modifications to food choices. Whilst food choices can be affected by a range of factors, including social, demographic, sensory, economic, cultural and behavioural, the ability to bite and chew is also important [2, 3]. Impaired masticatory ability has also been shown to be associated with reduced nutrient intake, poor nutritional status and subsequent health [4, 5].

The precise nature of the relationship between masticatory ability and food choice is not entirely clear. Population surveys have indicated that people with no natural teeth (edentate) choose foods which are higher in fat but lower in fibre, fruits and vegetables when compared with patients with natural teeth [6]. It might be expected that dental status would be directly associated with food choice and diet, but the evidence suggests that this is not a causal relationship. It has been shown that as natural teeth are lost, chewing function can be negatively affected but this may

© Springer Nature Switzerland AG 2021
G. McKenna (ed.), *Nutrition and Oral Health*, https://doi.org/10.1007/978-3-030-80526-5_7

occur slowly over time as patients adapt to their reduced masticatory ability [7].

Amongst older patients, chewing problems are relatively common. In a study of 1755 people aged 65 years and older, 13% with impaired dentitions said that they 'often' or 'always' had problems biting or chewing. Amongst the same group, 10% had experienced frequent limitations in the kinds or amounts of food eaten, whilst 9% always perceived discomfort whilst eating [8]. In another study, one in five older people reported that oral conditions prevented them from eating the foods they would like to choose, 15% took longer to complete their meal and their enjoyment of food was limited by oral conditions. In addition, 5% avoided eating with other people because of chewing problems. Edentulous subjects were more affected than dentate individuals [9]. Other studies have shown that patients with xerostomia, which affects about 20% of older people, also complained of difficulties eating certain foods [10].

7.1.2 Nutritional Status

Diet plays a key role in disease prevention in older age, as poor diet has been linked to illnesses such as osteoporosis, atherosclerosis and bowel disease. Poor oral health and loss of teeth can have very significant negative effects on dietary intake and nutritional status for older patients. In fact, the American Dietetic Association has stated that oral health and nutrition have a 'synergistic bidirectional relationship' [11]. The loss of natural teeth can alter older patients' selection of foods. When fewer natural teeth are present, older people tend to choose foods which are softer and easier to chew. However, these foods are often low in nutrients including fibre, high in calories and complex carbohydrates [12]. It has been shown that older patients' perceived ability to chew foods is closely associated with the number of natural teeth remaining [13]. In addition to the number of natural teeth remaining, the number of occluding pairs of teeth also appears to be very important [14].

In studies of nutrition in adult populations, poor-quality diet has been reported in adults missing natural teeth and wearing partial and complete dentures [15]. Some of the possible reasons for this are thought to be difficulty in chewing hard foods such as raw vegetables and fruits and a decreased sense of taste [16]. Conversely, there is some limited evidence that improvement of dentition and oral health generally has very positive effects on these parameters. The United Kingdom National Diet and Nutrition Survey of people aged 65 years and over reported on the oral health of the participants in the survey. A consistent finding in their report was that dentate individuals had higher daily intake of protein, fibre, calcium, iron and vitamin C than their edentulous counterparts [17, 18]. This has implications for general health in adults, as poor diet may lead to deficiency of nutrients and illnesses such as osteoporosis, atherosclerosis and bowel disease. Although there are many factors which influence food selection, it seems likely that preservation of a critical number of natural, disease-free teeth is a significant factor facilitating a healthy diet. These findings from the United Kingdom have been confirmed in other studies of frail elders including Finland and Brazil [19]. The risk of malnutrition in frail elders is such that Poulsen and co-workers have recently recommended that oral examination should form part of routine hospital admission procedures for geriatric admissions [20].

Markers of nutritional status can be found within the blood biochemistry of all patients and haematological samples have been used to measure nutritional status for a variety of patient groups. Nutrients including vitamin B12 and folate have been shown to decrease where malnutrition exists particularly in older patients. These vitamins are inextricably linked and deficiency can be caused by chronic generalised malabsorption or malnutrition. Deficiency of either vitamin can result in disruption of DNA synthesis caused by thymidine lack and resulting megaloblastic anaemia. In addition, deficiency of these vitamins can result in disturbances of methylation, leading to effects on the nervous system and other organs

[21]. Amongst many older populations, particularly those in Northern European countries, low levels of vitamin D have been reported as a marker of malnutrition. Poor vitamin D status has serious implications for the long-term risk of osteoporosis, and vitamin D status may negatively impact other chronic diseases such as cancer and cardiovascular disease. Probably the most widely reported nutritional markers of malnutrition are serum albumin and total cholesterol which are markers for protein energy malnutrition (PEM) [22]. Hypoalbuminaemia is found in more than 60% of malnourished geriatric patients, and albumin remains one of the most sensitive markers of malnutrition.

7.1.3 Quality of Life

Oral health is understood to be integral to both systemic health and overall quality of life. As such, the concept of oral health-related quality of life (OHrQoL) delineates how oral health outcomes impact an individual's overall quality of life [23]. The concept of OHrQoL captures all of the important aspects of oral health which contribute to quality of life including function (chewing, biting, speaking, swallowing), psychological factors (aesthetics, self-esteem, appearance), social factors (relating to interactions with others) and experience of pain and discomfort [24].

A systematic review and meta-analysis have indicated that loss of natural teeth is directly and negatively associated with OHrQoL [25]. Analysed evidence was derived from all parts of the world, including Europe, North and Southern America, Southeast Asia (China, Japan, South Korea, Sri Lanka) and Africa (Tanzania). This review included a study from Finland which used nationally representative population data sets to explore the relationship between age, tooth loss and OHrQoL. The authors reported that age and tooth loss are closely associated, but have independent effects on OHrQoL [26]. Tooth loss (which is associated with increasing age) is associated with more negative impacts, whilst increasing age independently results in fewer. In all of the populations and subpopulations studied, a complete or almost complete natural dentition was associated with the best OHrQoL.

Tooth loss not only impairs chewing functions, speech and appearance, but also negatively affects people's self-worth by hampering a person's sense of intactness and pride, as well as interpersonal relationships [27]. Prosthodontic replacement of missing teeth can also impact OHrQoL, with a generally positive impact reported for fixed prostheses compared with mixed impacts for removable prostheses [28, 29].

7.2 Tooth Replacement for Edentate Adults

7.2.1 Complete Replacement Dentures

For the majority of edentate patients, missing natural teeth are replaced with complete replacement dentures (Fig. 7.1). These removable prostheses are designed to replace the teeth as well as the hard and soft tissues which previously supported them [30]. A variety of methods can be utilised to construct the prostheses, including modern methods based on CAD-CAM technology, but all produce a similar final result of replacement teeth and the associated hard and soft tissues [31]. Construction of high-quality complete replacement dentures can have positive impacts on a variety of important factors including aesthetics, speech and phonics, and quality of

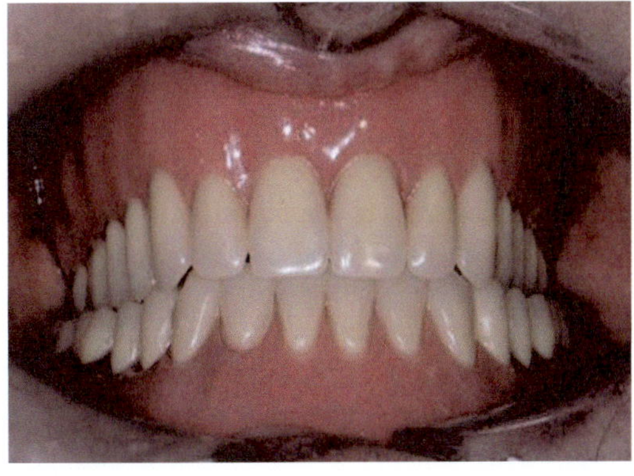

Fig. 7.1 Complete upper and lower complete replacement dentures

life [32–34]. Whilst these outcomes are very important, one of the main functions of complete replacement dentures is to facilitate mastication. However, evidence suggests that providing complete replacement dentures alone has very limited positive impact on the nutritional status for older adults. In a study of patients within a residential care home, Wostmann et al. demonstrated that provision of new complete dentures had a positive impact on masticatory ability measured using a masticatory efficiency test (MET). However, no improvements in nutritional status were noted according to haematological measures or the Mini Nutritional Assessment (MNA) [35].

In comparison, an increasing body of evidence supports the combination of tooth replacement using complete dentures and a dietary intervention component amongst this population group. Studies have demonstrated improvements in dietary intake after this intervention ranging from increases in fruits and vegetables to proteins [36]. In a randomised controlled clinical trial of edentate older adults in Japan, all patients within the study received new complete dentures. The intervention group within the study (n = 35) also received concurrent dietary advice based on information from the Japanese Food Guide. Patients within the intervention group recorded significantly higher intakes of nutrients including protein, magnesium and vitamin B1 [37].

7.2.2 Implant-Supported Prostheses

Oral rehabilitation with implant-supported prostheses has become a well-documented therapy for edentate older adults, particularly in the lower arch (Fig. 7.2) [38]. Numerous studies have proven the benefits of implant-retained overdenture treatment for edentulous patients including improvements in OHrQoL and masticatory function which exceed those offered by complete replacement dentures [39, 40].

Given that implant-retained prostheses are regarded as superior to conventional complete dentures due to improved stability and comfort, a number of studies have also investigated their impact on nutritional parameters [41, 42]. One

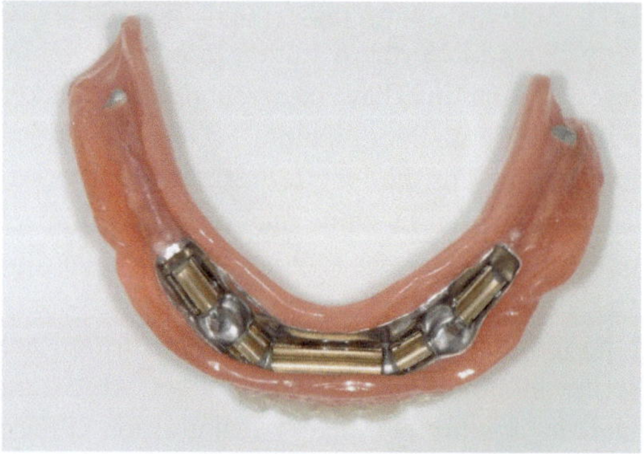

Fig. 7.2 A lower implant-supported overdenture for an edentate patient

study recruited 255 independently living edentate adults aged 65 years and older in Montreal, Canada. The participants were randomly assigned to two treatment groups using block randomisation, where patients received either a complete conventional lower denture or a two-implant-retained lower overdenture. The outcome measure reported was the impact of prosthodontic rehabilitation on dietary intake. Patients self-reported food intake using a 24 dietary recall method at baseline and again 12 months after treatment intervention. Dietary intake values were used to calculate intake of dietary fibre, macronutrients (proteins, fat and carbohydrates), micronutrients (vitamins A, B6, B12, C and D; thiamine; riboflavin; folate; and niacin) and energy. Statistical analysis revealed no significant between-group differences in terms of intake of dietary fibre, energy, macronutrients or micronutrients at either baseline or 12 months after prosthodontic intervention [43]. As with complete replacement dentures it would appear that prosthodontic implant treatment alone has very limited positive impact on the nutritional status for older adults [44].

7.3 Tooth Replacement for Partially Dentate Adults

7.3.1 Removable Partial Dentures

For partially dentate older adults the majority of patients currently receive removable partial dentures (RPDs) to replace missing teeth (Fig. 7.3).

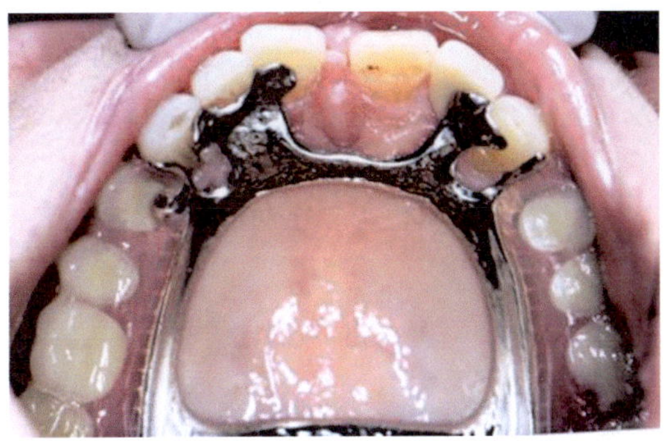

Fig. 7.3 Removable upper partial denture

Impact on OHrQoL has been used as an outcome measure to indicate the effect of replacing missing natural teeth for a variety of patient groups. In partially dentate patients, improvement in OHrQoL after replacement of teeth with RPDs can be difficult to demonstrate consistently [45]. In a study of 60 patients with missing posterior teeth half the participants received RPDs. These patients indicated a significant improvement in satisfaction 3 months and 1 year after treatment intervention [46]. A more recent study has also indicated significant improvements in OHrQoL for patients restored using RPDs. Although a pilot study, 17 patients indicated a significant improvement in Oral Health Impact Profile (OHIP) scores 6 weeks, 6 months and 12 months after treatment [47]. However, other studies have indicated that patients often only appear to perceive meaningful benefits from RPDs when anterior teeth are replaced resulting in many patients never or only occasionally wearing the RPDs constructed [48, 49].

Evidence does suggest that provision of RPDs can elicit a significant improvement in masticatory performance in partially dentate patients. A study by Wallace et al. recruited partially dentate older patients and measured masticatory performance before and after denture construction using a validated colour-mixing ability test [50]. In addition to measuring masticatory performance, the study also collected information on nutritional status using biochemical markers and the Mini Nutritional Assessment (MNA). The study demonstrated that after RPD construction, masticatory performance increased significantly as the participants were provided with more prosthetic teeth to chew with. However, nutritional status did not improve in line with masticatory performance. The authors concluded that improvements in masticatory performance, generated through replacing missing natural teeth, may only have minor associations with nutritional status amongst partially dentate patients [50].

7.3.2 Functionally Orientated Tooth Replacement

Given patients' dislike of RPDs, their biological cost and high levels of non-compliance, other treatment options should be considered when planning tooth replacement for older, partially dentate patients [51]. Some researchers have suggested that older adults have different functional needs to young patients and therefore do not need a complete natural dentition. The shortened dental arch concept (SDA) has been successfully implemented in older patients by preserving anterior teeth in preference to molars which are more difficult to maintain [52].

Käyser first described the SDA as 'a dentition where the most posterior teeth are missing' [52]. The molar regions play important roles in mastication and stabilisation; however they are high-risk teeth for caries and periodontal disease, and possibilities for restorative treatment are often limited. The concept of the SDA involves the direction of treatment efforts and resources towards preservation of the anterior and premolar teeth, which Käyser and Witter suggest are the 'strategic' part of the dental arch [53]. In practical terms, however, it is impossible to maintain a natural shortened dental arch for all patients as some will have suffered trauma or extensive disease to their anterior teeth, resulting in tooth loss and the need for prosthetic replacement. In order to conform to the principles of the SDA, replacement of missing teeth should be provided using fixed prosthodontics. Especially in partially reduced dentitions with (almost) sound remaining teeth adhesive bridgework offers a predictable means of replacing missing teeth [54, 55]. Adhesive bridges are relatively easy to place and

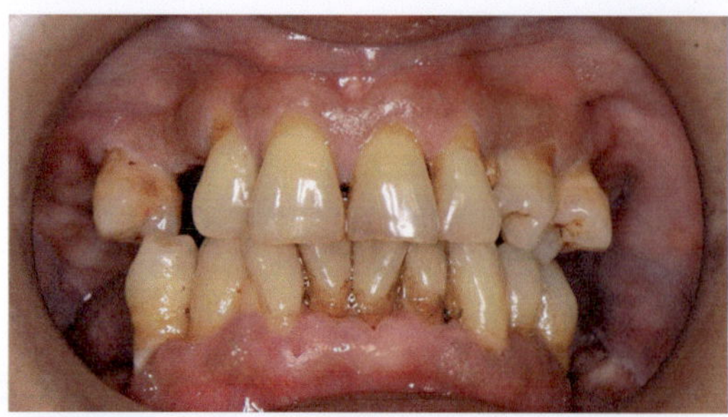

Fig. 7.4 Patient with a functional SDA

well accepted by the patient plus their biological price is low compared to conventional bridges and RPDs [56, 57].

Käyser found sufficient oral function in a SDA when at least four occlusal units remained, preferably in a symmetrical position (Fig. 7.4). According to the same author, fewer than 12 front teeth and 8 premolars result in a SDA with impaired oral function [52]. Sarita and co-workers found that chewing ability decreased as occluding pairs of teeth decreased [58]. They found that a SDA with intact premolar regions and at least one occluding pair of molars provided sufficient chewing ability, and that a SDA comprising 20 teeth (intact anterior region and four pairs of occluding posterior teeth) can provide satisfactory chewing ability for soft foods but not all hard foods. In a study comparing subjects with a complete dental arch, interrupted dental arches and SDA, Montero et al. found that the impact of arch length on oral functionality was proportional to the number of absent occlusal units [59].

The impact of functional replacement of missing teeth using the principles of the SDA on nutritional outcomes has been studied, most notably in a randomised controlled clinical trial by McKenna et al. [60]. This study compared tooth replacement treatment using RPDs with the SDA approach and demonstrated superiority for functionally orientated treatment according to quality of life and cost-effectiveness outcomes [61, 62]. Impact on nutritional status was measured using the Mini Nutritional Assessment (MNA) and a series of haematological biomarkers including serum folate, ferritin and albumin [63]. Despite a comprehensive assessment, whilst replacement of missing teeth according to a func-

tionally orientated approach demonstrated improvements in chewing function, it did not demonstrate a consistent improvement in nutritional status [50, 64].

7.4 Conclusion

Whilst it is clear that oral health status, particularly related to numbers of teeth, plays an important role in masticatory function for older adults, it is less clear that prosthodontic treatment alone to replace missing teeth has a positive impact on nutritional status. A consistent finding from research into all prosthodontic treatment modalities used to rehabilitate edentate and partially dentate patients was that tooth replacement alone was insufficient to engender dietary changes. It would appear that nutritional counselling alongside prosthodontic interventions offers a more promising approach. This would suggest that patients undergoing prosthodontic treatment to replace missing teeth should also receive nutritional counselling from either their dentist or a dietician if improvements in nutritional status are to be achieved.

References

1. Boretti G, Bickel M, Geering AH. A review of masticatory ability and efficiency. J Prosthet Dent. 1995;74(4):400–3. https://doi.org/10.1016/S0022-3913(05)80381-6.
2. Sheiham A, Steele J, Marcenes W, et al. The relationship among dental status, nutrient intake, and nutritional status in older people. J Dent Res. 2001;80(2):408–13. https://doi.org/10.1177/00220345010800020201.
3. Sheiham A, Steele J. Does the condition of the mouth and teeth affect the ability to eat certain foods, nutrient and dietary intake and nutritional status amongst older people? Public Health Nutr. 2001;4(3):797–803. https://doi.org/10.1079/phn2000116.
4. Joshipura KJ, Rimm EB, Douglass CW, Trichopoulos D, Ascherio A, Willett WC. Poor oral health and coronary heart disease. J Dent Res. 1996;75(9):1631–6. https://doi.org/10.1177/00220345960750090301.
5. Mathews MJ, Mathews EH, Mathews GE. Oral health and coronary heart disease. BMC Oral Health. 2016;16(1):122. https://doi.org/10.1186/s12903-016-0316-7.

6. Sheiham A, Steele JG, Marcenes W, Finch S, Walls AW. The impact of oral health on stated ability to eat certain foods; findings from the National Diet and Nutrition Survey of Older People in Great Britain. Gerodontology. 1999;16(1):11–20. https://doi.org/10.1111/j.1741-2358.1999.00011.x.

7. Brennan DS, Spencer AJ, Roberts-Thomson KF. Tooth loss, chewing ability and quality of life. Qual Life Res. 2008;17(2):227–35. https://doi.org/10.1007/s11136-007-9293-2.

8. Atchison K, Dolan T. Development of the Geriatric Oral Health Assessment Index. J Dent Educ. 1990;54(11):680–7. https://doi.org/10.1002/j.0022-0337.1990.54.11.tb02481.x.

9. Locker D. The burden of oral disorders in a population of older adults. Community Dent Health. 1992;9(2):109–24.

10. Locker D. Subjective reports of oral dryness in an older adult population. Community Dent Oral Epidemiol. 1993;21(3):165–8. https://doi.org/10.1111/j.1600-0528.1993.tb00744.x.

11. Touger-Decker R, Mobley C. Position of the Academy of Nutrition and Dietetics: Oral Health and Nutrition. J Acad Nutr Diet. 2013;113(5):693–701. https://doi.org/10.1016/j.jand.2013.03.001.

12. Moynihan PJ, Mulvaney CE, Adamson AJ, et al. The nutrition knowledge of older adults living in sheltered housing accommodation. J Hum Nutr Diet. 2007;20(5):446–58. https://doi.org/10.1111/j.1365-277X.2007.00808.x.

13. Papas AS. Relationships among education, dentate status, and diet in adults. Spec Care Dent. 1998;18(1):26–32. https://doi.org/10.1111/j.1754-4505.1998.tb01355.x.

14. Leake JL. An Index of Chewing Ability. J Public Health Dent. 1990;50(4):262–7. https://doi.org/10.1111/j.1752-7325.1990.tb02133.x.

15. Sheiham A, Steele JG, Marcenes W, Tsakos G, Finch S, Walls AWG. Prevalence of impacts of dental and oral disorders and their effects on eating among older people, a national survey in Great Britain. Community Dent Oral Epidemiol. 2001;29(3):195–203. https://doi.org/10.1034/j.1600-0528.2001.290305.x.

16. McKenna G, Burke FM. Age-related oral changes. Dent Update. 2010;37(8):519–23. https://doi.org/10.12968/denu.2010.37.8.519.

17. Steele J. National diet and nutrition survey: people aged 65 years and over. Report of the Oral Health Survey. Vol 2, 1998.

18. Watson S, McGowan L, McCrum L-A, et al. The impact of dental status on perceived ability to eat certain foods and nutrient intakes in older adults: cross-sectional analysis of the UK National Diet and Nutrition Survey 2008-2014. Int J Behav Nutr Phys Act. 2019;16(1):43. https://doi.org/10.1186/s12966-019-0803-8.

19. De Marchi RJ, Hugo FN, Padilha DMP, et al. Edentulism, use of dentures and consumption of fruit and vegetables in south Brazilian community-dwelling elderly. J Oral Rehabil. 2011;38(7):533–40. https://doi.org/10.1111/j.1365-2842.2010.02189.x.

20. Poulsen I, Rahm Hallberg I, Schroll M. Nutritional status and associated factors on geriatric admission. J Nutr Heal Aging. 2006;10(2):84–90.

21. Varela-Moreiras G, Murphy MM, Scott JM. Cobalamin, folic acid, and homocysteine. Nutr Rev. 2009;67:S69–72. https://doi.org/10.1111/j.1753-4887.2009.00163.x.

22. Omran ML, Morley JE. Assessment of protein energy malnutrition in older persons, part I: History, examination, body composition, and screening tools. Nutrition. 2000;16(1):50–63. https://doi.org/10.1016/S0899-9007(99)00224-5.

23. Baiju R, Peter E, Varghese N, Sivaram R. Oral health and quality of life: current concepts. J Clin Diagnostic Res. 2017;11(6):ZE21–6. https://doi.org/10.7860/JCDR/2017/25866.10110.

24. Locker D. Oral health and quality of life. Oral Health Prev Dent. 2004;2004:247–53. https://doi.org/10.3290/j.ohpd.a10161.

25. Gerritsen AE, Allen PF, Witter DJ, Bronkhorst EM, Creugers NHJ. Tooth loss and oral health-related quality of life: A systematic review and meta-analysis. Health Qual Life Outcomes. 2010;8:126. https://doi.org/10.1186/1477-7525-8-126.

26. Lahti S, Suominen-Taipale L, Hausen H. Oral health impacts among adults in Finland: Competing effects of age, number of teeth, and removable dentures. Eur J Oral Sci. 2008;116(3):260–6. https://doi.org/10.1111/j.1600-0722.2008.00540.x.

27. Niesten D, Van Mourik K, Van Der Sanden W. The impact of having natural teeth on the QoL of frail dentulous older people: a qualitative study. BMC Public Health. 2012;12:839. https://doi.org/10.1186/1471-2458-12-839.

28. Ali Z, Baker SR, Shahrbaf S, Martin N, Vettore MV. Oral health-related quality of life after prosthodontic treatment for patients with partial edentulism: A systematic review and meta-analysis. J Prosthet Dent. 2019;121(1):59–68. https://doi.org/10.1016/j.prosdent.2018.03.003.

29. McLister C, Donnelly M, Cardwell CR, et al. Effectiveness of prosthodontic interventions and survival of remaining teeth in adult patients with shortened dental arches—a systematic review. J Dent. 2018;78:31–9. https://doi.org/10.1016/j.jdent.2018.02.003.

30. Srinivasan M, Schimmel M, Leles C, McKenna G. Managing Edentate Older Adults. Prim Dent J. 2020;9(3):29–33. https://doi.org/10.1177/2050168420943410.

31. Srinivasan M, Schimmel M, Naharro M, O'Neill C, McKenna G, Müller F. CAD/CAM milled removable complete dentures: time and cost estimation study. J Dent. 2019;80:75–9. https://doi.org/10.1016/j.jdent.2018.09.003.

32. Nuñez MCO, Silva DC, Barcelos BA, Leles CR. Patient satisfaction and oral health-related quality of life after treatment with traditional and simplified protocols for complete denture construction. Gerodontology. 2015;32(4):247–53. https://doi.org/10.1111/ger.12078.

33. Ellis JS, Pelekis ND, Thomason JM. Conventional rehabilitation of edentulous patients: the impact on oral health-related quality of life and patient satisfaction. J Prosthodont. 2007;16(1):37–42. https://doi.org/10.1111/j.1532-849X.2006.00152.x.

34. Hsu YJ, Lin JR, Hsu JF. Patient satisfaction, clinical outcomes and oral health-related quality of life after treatment with traditional and modified protocols for complete dentures. J Dent Sci. 2021;32(4):247–53. https://doi.org/10.1016/j.jds.2020.05.024.

35. Wöstmann B, Michel K, Brinkert B, Melchheier-Weskott A, Rehmann P, Balkenhol M. Influence of denture improvement on the nutritional status and quality of life of geriatric patients. J Dent. 2008;36(10):816–21. https://doi.org/10.1016/j.jdent.2008.05.017.

36. Bradbury J, Thomason JM, Jepson NJA, Walls AWG, Allen PF, Moynihan PJ. Nutrition counseling increases fruit and vegetable intake in the edentulous. J Dent Res. 2006;85(5):463–8. https://doi.org/10.1177/154405910608500513.

37. Amagai N, Komagamine Y, Kanazawa M, et al. The effect of prosthetic rehabilitation and simple dietary counseling on food intake and oral health related quality of life among the edentulous individuals: a randomized controlled trial. J Dent. 2017;65:89–94. https://doi.org/10.1016/j.jdent.2017.07.011.

38. Schimmel M, Srinivasan M, McKenna G, Müller F. Effect of advanced age and/or systemic medical conditions on dental implant survival: a systematic review and meta-analysis. Clin Oral Implants Res. 2018;29:311–30. https://doi.org/10.1111/clr.13288.

39. Rashid F, Awad MA, Thomason JM, et al. The effectiveness of 2-implant overdentures - a pragmatic international multicentre study. J Oral Rehabil. 2011;38(3):176–84. https://doi.org/10.1111/j.1365-2842.2010.02143.x.

40. Allen PF, Thomason JM, Jepson NJA, Nohl F, Smith DG, Ellis J. A randomized controlled trial of implant-retained mandibular overdentures. J Dent Res. 2006;85(6):547–51. https://doi.org/10.1177/154405910608500613.

41. Thomason JM, Feine J, Exley C, et al. Mandibular two implant-supported overdentures as the first choice standard of care for edentulous patients - the York consensus statement. Br Dent J. 2009;207(4):185–6. https://doi.org/10.1038/sj.bdj.2009.728.

42. Feine JS, Carlsson GE, Awad MA, et al. The McGill consensus statement on overdentures. Mandibular two-implant overdentures as first choice standard of care for edentulous patients. Gerodontology. 2002;19(1):3–4. https://doi.org/10.1111/j.1741-2358.2002.00003.x.

43. Hamdan NM, Gray-Donald K, Awad MA, Johnson-Down L, Wollin S, Feine JS. Do implant overdentures improve dietary intake? A randomized clinical trial. J Dent Res. 2013;92:146S–53S. https://doi.org/10.1177/0022034513504948.

44. McKenna G. Implant-retained overdentures did not have a significant improvement in dietary intake. Evid Based Dent. 2014;15(3):89. https://doi.org/10.1038/sj.ebd.6401048.

45. Mericske-Stern R. Removable Partial Dentures. Int J Prosthodont. 2009;22(5):508–11.

46. Jepson NJA, Allen PF, Moynihan P, Peter K, Thomason JM. Patient satisfaction following restoration of shortened mandibular dental arches in a randomized controlled trial. Int J Prosthodont. 2003;16(4):409–14.

47. Wolfart S, Heydecke G, Luthardt RG, et al. Effects of prosthetic treatment for shortened dental arches on oral health-related quality of life, self-reports of pain and jaw disability: Results from the pilot-phase of a randomized multicentre trial. J Oral Rehabil. 2005;32(11):815–22. https://doi.org/10.1111/j.1365-2842.2005.01522.x.

48. Jepson NJ, Thomason JM, Steele JG. The influence of denture design on patient acceptance of partial dentures. Br Dent J. 1995;178(8):296–300. https://doi.org/10.1038/sj.bdj.4808742.

49. Allen F. Factors influencing the provision of removable partial dentures by dentists in Ireland. J Ir Dent Assoc. 2010;56(5):224–9.

50. Wallace S, Samietz S, Abbas M, McKenna G, Woodside JV, Schimmel M. Impact of prosthodontic rehabilitation on the masticatory performance of partially dentate older patients: can it predict nutritional state? Results from a RCT. J Dent. 2018;68:66–71. https://doi.org/10.1016/j.jdent.2017.11.003.

51. Allen PF, McKenna G, Creugers N. Prosthodontic care for elderly patients. Dent Update. 2011;38(7):460–2. https://doi.org/10.12968/denu.2011.38.7.460.

52. Kayser AF. Shortened dental arches and oral function. J Oral Rehabil. 1981;8(5):457–62. https://doi.org/10.1111/j.1365-2842.1981.tb00519.x.

53. Kayser A, Witter DJ. Oral functional needs and its consequences for dentulous older people. Community Dent Health. 1985;2(4):285–91.

54. Jepson NJA, Allen PF. Short and sticky options in the treatment of the partially dentate patient. Br Dent J. 1999;187(12):646–52. https://doi.org/10.1038/sj.bdj.4800357a.

55. McKenna G, Tada S, McLister C, et al. Tooth replacement options for partially dentate older adults: a survival analysis. J Dent. 2020;103:103468. https://doi.org/10.1016/j.jdent.2020.103468.

56. Budtz-Jørgensen E, Isidor F. A 5-year longitudinal study of cantilevered fixed partial dentures compared with removable partial dentures in a geriatric population. J Prosthet Dent. 1990;64(1):42–7. https://doi.org/10.1016/0022-3913(90)90151-2.

57. Jepson NJA, Moynihan RJ, Kelly PJ, Watson GW, Thomason JM. Caries incidence following restoration of shortened lower dental arches in a randomized controlled trial. Br Dent J. 2001;191(3):140–4. https://doi.org/10.1038/sj.bdj.4801122a.

58. Sarita PTN, Witter DJ, Kreulen CM, Van't Hof MA, Creugers NHJ. Chewing ability of subjects with shortened dental arches. Community Dent Oral Epidemiol. 2003;31(5):328–34. https://doi.org/10.1034/j.1600-0528.2003.t01-1-00011.x.

59. Montero J, Bravo M, Hernández LA, Dib A. Effect of arch length on the functional well-being of dentate adults. J Oral Rehabil. 2009;36(5):338–45. https://doi.org/10.1111/j.1365-2842.2009.01945.x.

60. McKenna G, Allen PF, O'Mahony D, Cronin M, Damata C, Woods N. The impact of rehabilitation using removable partial dentures and functionally orientated treatment on oral health-related quality of life: a randomised controlled clinical trial. J Dent. 2015;43(1):66–71. https://doi.org/10.1016/j.jdent.2014.06.006.

61. McKenna G, Allen PF, Hayes M, DaMata C, Moore C, Cronin M. Impact of oral rehabilitation on the quality of life of partially dentate elders in a randomized controlled clinical trial: 2 year follow-up. PLoS One. 2018;13(10):e0203349. https://doi.org/10.1371/journal.pone.0203349.

62. McKenna G, Allen F, Woods N, et al. Cost-effectiveness of tooth replacement strategies for partially dentate elderly: a randomized controlled clinical trial. Community Dent Oral Epidemiol. 2014;42(4):366–74. https://doi.org/10.1111/cdoe.12085.

63. McKenna G, Allen PF, Flynn A, et al. Impact of tooth replacement strategies on the nutritional status of partially-dentate elders. Gerodontology. 2012;29(2):e883–90. https://doi.org/10.1111/j.1741-2358.2011.00579.x.

64. McKenna G, Allen PF, O'Mahony D, Cronin M, DaMata C, Woods N. Impact of tooth replacement on the nutritional status of partially dentate elders. Clin Oral Investig. 2015;19(8):1991–8. https://doi.org/10.1007/s00784-015-1409-4.

Strategies for Changing Dietary Behaviour

8

Laura McGowan

Abstract

Globally, diets are suboptimal for health amongst both adults and children. In Western societies in particular, there is an overconsumption of foods high in fat, salt and sugar, coupled with inadequate intakes of fibre, wholegrains, fruits and vegetables, and fish. Linked to poor-quality dietary intake, there has also been a significant increase in levels of obesity, with rates tripling in adults in the United Kingdom in the past 20 years. This has led to an increase in obesity-related comorbidities such as type 2 diabetes, cardiovascular disease and certain cancers. There is consensus amongst experts that long-term, effective diet and lifestyle changes are needed to improve population health, alongside substantial changes to social and environmental drivers within the food system. Significant advances have been made in the field of behavioural science in the past decade, with greater shared understanding of the important strategies and techniques which can be used in the design of interventions to change dietary behaviour amongst adults.

L. McGowan (✉)
Centre for Public Health, School of Medicine, Dentistry and Biomedical Sciences, Queen's University Belfast, Belfast, United Kingdom

Institute for Global Food Security, School of Biological Sciences, Queen's University Belfast, Belfast, United Kingdom
e-mail: laura.mcgowan@qub.ac.uk

Whilst this chapter predominantly highlights evidence-based strategies which can be implemented to effect positive dietary changes in adults on an individual level, it is not without acknowledgement of the pivotal role played by wider societal and environmental influences coupled with psychological and biological repsonses driving food intake. From policymakers and legislation to health professionals and healthcare services, and to the role of the individual, all components are of critical importance in order to bring about long-term positive dietary changes.

8.1 Current Dietary Patterns in Adults

'Diet evolves over time, being influenced by many social and economic factors that interact in a complex manner to shape individual dietary patterns' [1].

It is now the case that globally, people are consuming more foods high in energy, fats, free sugars and salt/sodium, and many people do not eat enough fruits, vegetables and other dietary fibre such as wholegrains to benefit health [1]. The National Diet and Nutrition Survey Rolling Programme (NDNS RP) is a repeated, cross-sectional survey designed to assess the dietary habits and nutritional status of adults and children in the United Kingdom. Since 2008, the NDNS has run continuously covering a representative sample of both adults and children, and allows for detailed diet and nutritional analyses for a range of age groups. Public Health England published the NDNS Report of Years 9 to 11 (combined) of the Rolling Programme (2016/2017–2018/2019) in December 2020 which illustrated that overall, the UK population continues to consume too much sugar and saturated fat, and not enough fruits, vegetables, oily fish and fibre [2]. Intakes of free sugars, saturated fats and fibre failed to meet the recommendations for a healthy diet in all age groups [2]. For example, only 33% of adults aged 19–64 years, 40% of older adults aged 65–74 years and 27% of adults aged over 75 years meet the UK recommendations to consume at least five portions of fruits and vegetables per day [2, 3]. Regarding fibre, mean intakes were below the recommendation of 30 g/day in all adults, often falling short by as much as 10–14 g/day [2]. Fruits and vegetables (FV) are of particular significance for protecting health, especially in ageing adults, wherein adequate intake of FV has been associated with a lower risk of all-cause mortality, particularly cardiovascular mortality [4]. More recently, the health-protective effects of fibre have been shown in a large-scale systematic review and meta-analysis of over 185 prospective studies and 58 clinical trials, where clear benefits to health were noted from relatively high intakes of dietary fibre and wholegrains [5]. The authors suggested that recommendations to increase dietary fibre intake and to replace refined grains with wholegrains should be a public health focus as it is expected to benefit health [5].

8.1.1 Diet and Obesity

Whilst the drivers regarding the development of obesity are extremely complex and multifactorial [6] (see Fig. 8.1), dietary intake plays a central role in the energy balance equation (i.e. energy in or 'calories ingested' versus energy expended or 'calories used up'). Obesity has been defined as 'a chronic relapsing medical condition' which may impair health, result in unwarranted stigma and increase mortality rates [7, 8]. In most cases,

the development of obesity is linked to an increased caloric intake (over and above energy expenditure) or positive energy balance over a period of time [9]. However, the drivers of this increased caloric intake can be considered part of a complex biological-psychological-social and economic model, with many individuals predisposed to obesity (or thinness) as a result of their genetic make-up [10, 11].

Levels of obesity in the United Kingdom (and beyond) remain a public health concern, with approximately one in four adults over 16 years considered to have obesity (body mass index (BMI) of 30 kg/m^2 or more) [12]. Obesity rates in the United Kingdom peak around the ages of 55–64 years (37.3% for men, 34% for women) with only a slight decline seen in the over 75 years age group [12]. As noted, there are many reasons for increasing levels of obesity including increasingly sedentary lifestyles coupled with the abundance of cheap, highly palatable, energy-dense but often nutrient-poor ultra-processed food [6]. Indeed, some individuals are also predisposed to have greater difficulties navigating the 'obesogenic' environment due to their biological make-up (i.e. genetics), where differences in appetite and the reward gained from food vary greatly between individuals [11]. An EAT-Lancet commission in 2019 further highlighted the *global syndemic of obesity, undernutrition and climate change'* suggesting that a radical rethink of how we 'eat, live, consume and move' is needed in order to have any chance of improving human health [8]. Yet, even in the face of the complex drivers of food choice, individuals and individual-behaviour still matter, given that we make multiple decisions each day regarding our food and activity behaviour within our own contexts and environments [13]. This chapter highlights the evidence base surrounding one element of this complex system, focusing on the role for individual behaviour change in adults.

8.1.2 Need for Behaviour Change

In ageing adults, the increasing loss of natural teeth has been shown to significantly reduce chewing performance and consequently act as a

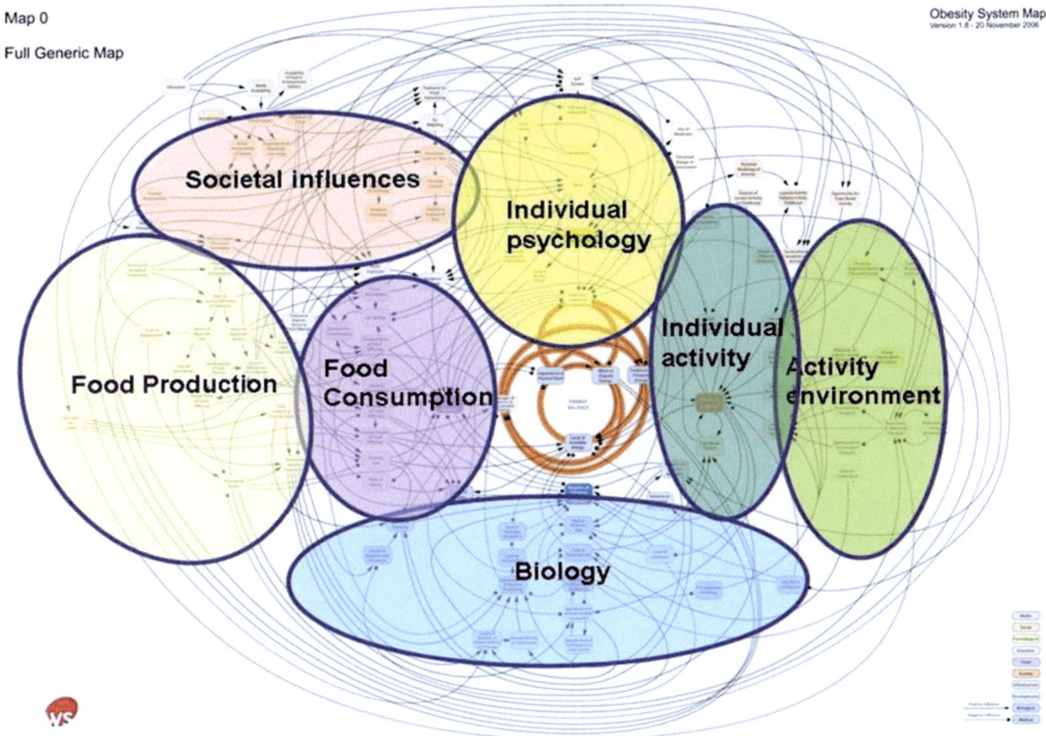

Fig. 8.1 Obesity System Map [6]

significant barrier to healthy food choices [14]. Adults who encounter such difficulties are at greater risk of having a poor-quality diet, as they are less likely to opt for nutrient-dense foods that are harder to masticate such as fruits, vegetables or fibre-rich foods. Instead, they replace them with easier-to-chew foods, which are often lacking in key nutrients, and of a high calorie and low dietary fibre content [15–17]. This is of particular concern given that levels of obesity tend to peak during this life stage [12]. Existing randomized controlled trials (RCT) evidence has shown that replacing missing teeth alone (using a variety of oral rehabilitation methods) and not targeting diet is not consistently predictive of wide-ranging dietary changes which might lead to an improvement in objective nutritional status, e.g. via haematological markers [18, 19]. This highlights an opportunity for targeted or purposeful dietary intervention in order to address diet and nutritional challenges in this growing population group [20].

8.2 Advancing the Science of Behaviour Change

Historically, interventions designed to bring about change in behaviour, and particularly in complex dietary behaviour, have been poorly described in the published literature. The theoretical underpinnings, strategies or techniques that have been employed in a study to bring about behaviour change have been difficult to disentangle, leading many to refer to the 'black box' of public health interventions [21]. Furthermore, the form of delivery (FoD) (i.e. who delivers the intervention, what it entails, where it is delivered, how often) and effectiveness are of known importance in complex behavioural interventions, yet often this level of detail is lacking in the published literature, limiting the ability to replicate interventions and identify effective intervention components [22, 23].

To ameliorate this, in 2008 the first consensually agreed taxonomy of theory-linked behaviour change techniques (BCTs) used in behaviour change interventions was published [24]. A BCT can be considered the 'active ingredient' or strategy in an intervention which is used to facilitate behaviour change. The defining characteristics of a BCT are that it is observable, replicable, irreducible, a component of an intervention designed to change behaviour and a postulated active ingredient within the intervention [25].

Production of this 26-item taxonomy was a pivotal moment in the field of behaviour change; the authors produced a set of theory-linked standardized definitions of the techniques and strategies included in behaviour change interventions to bring about change [24]. It was hoped that this 'common language' would facilitate the replication of effective behaviour change interventions and help to demystify the techniques contributing to intervention effectiveness (see Table 8.1 for examples of BCTs). Michie et al. (2011) then built upon this original taxonomy with a refined 40-item CALO-RE taxonomy in 2011, which focused specifically on techniques and strategies used to change behaviour in diet and physical activity (considered complex) interventions [26]. They created a list of 40 BCTs which could be used to characterize and describe the active components of inventions (for example, goal-setting and self-monitoring; see Table 8.1 for examples) to understand 'what works' in a given circum-stance, or within a particular population group in an intervention, thus maximizing future intervention efficacy [26, 27]. Currently, there are a number of taxonomies which have been created for different domains of behaviour change, with the most comprehensive to date being the BCT v1 Taxonomy, 93-item list of hierarchically structured BCTs [28].

8.3 Evidence-Based Strategies for Changing Diet

It has been illustrated that the inclusion of identifiable BCTs in an intervention is associated with greater efficacy across a range of health behaviour change interventions, including dietary improvements for adults of retirement age [29–31]. BCTs of importance with regard to adult dietary behaviour change interventions appear to relate to effective goal-setting and self-monitoring of behaviour [32], both core tenets of control theory [33] where setting a goal/objective and monitoring progress towards it are operating in a constant feedback loop. Dombrowski and colleagues conducted a systematic review and meta-analysis of multicomponent (complex) behaviour change interventions to address overweight and obesity in adults (average age 55 years) using the CALO-RE taxonomy [26] to code interventions.

Table 8.1 Illustrative selection of BCTs commonly found within behaviour change interventions [24]

Behaviour change technique (BCT)	Definition
1. Provide information about behaviour-health link	Provide general information about behavioural risk, e.g. susceptibility to poor health outcomes or mortality risk in relation to the behaviour
2. Provide information on consequences	Provide information about the benefits and costs of action or inaction, focusing on what will happen if the person does/does not perform the behaviour
3. Provide information about others' approval	Provide information about what others think about the person's behaviour and whether others will approve or disapprove of any proposed behaviour change
4. Prompt intention formation	Encouraging the person to decide to act or set a general goal, e.g. to make a behavioural resolution such as 'I will take more exercise next week'
5. Set graded tasks	Set easy tasks, and increase difficulty until target behaviour is performed
6. Model/demonstrate the behaviour	An expert shows the person how to correctly perform a behaviour, e.g. in class or on video
7. Prompt specific goal-setting	Involves detailed planning of what the person will do including a definition of the behaviour specifying frequency, intensity or duration as well as specification of at least one context, i.e. where, when, how or with whom
8. Prompt self-monitoring of behaviour	The person is asked to keep a record of specified behaviour/s (e.g. in a diary)

This research illustrated, using meta-regression, that including an increasing numbers of BCTs was not necessarily associated with better intervention outcomes, and that the specific BCTs 'provision of instructions', 'self-monitoring of behaviour', 'relapse prevention' and 'prompting practice' were linked to more successful lifestyle interventions (from 44 studies included in the review) [32].

Following this, Lara and colleagues conducted a secondary analysis of a systematic review and meta-analysis focusing on complex dietary interventions conducted with adults of retirement age, also coding intervention content and BCTs using the 40-item CALO-RE taxonomy [26, 30]. They examined BCTs used alongside intervention effectiveness outcomes, i.e. changes in participants' fruit and vegetable intake [30]. Of 22 papers included in the review, they identified 28 of the 40 BCTs contained within the CALO-RE taxonomy [26], with a median of 6 BCTs identified per dietary behaviour change intervention. Further analysis showed that interventions containing the BCTs 'barrier identification/problem solving' and 'plan social support/social change' led to the greatest change in FV intake compared to interventions not using these BCTs, equating to an average of one additional portion of FV per day (one portion of FV considered as approximately 80 g in the United Kingdom). Other BCTs of importance for positive changes in FV intake were 'goal-setting (outcome)', 'use of follow-up prompts' and 'provide feedback on performance', which also contributed towards an average increase of 39–66 g per day in FV consumption. Meta-regression showed that inclusion of one additional BCT led to an 8.3 g increase in FV intake. There was also a trend for greater FV intake gains in the dietary behaviour change interventions which were explicitly based upon theory (n = 14), although this did not reach statistical significance. The findings led the authors to conclude that the BCTs identified in this study may be 'active ingredients' for effectively increasing FV intake in adults of retirement age [30].

A systematic review conducted by McGowan and colleagues synthesized literature relating specifically to oral rehabilitation coupled with dietary intervention in adults, examining BCTs within interventions using the extended 93-item v1 BCT taxonomy [28, 34]. Of the nine studies included in the review, only two were theory based (n = 2) and BCTs and methods of delivery were poorly described within the published papers. Identifiable BCTs within the dietary behaviour change interventions ranged from one to nine (median n = 5), much like the review by Lara et al., with five interventions including tailored/personalized dietary information [30, 34]. The most common BCT identified across all studies was 'giving information on the health consequences of diet (in general)'. This latter type of information-giving strategy is not typically associated with the most effective behaviour change outcomes in this age group [30]. In one RCT included in the review involving theory-based, tailored dietary advice, participants in the dietary intervention group increased their FV intake by over 200 g/day (considered to be over two UK-sized FV portions) compared to the 'standard denture care' control group, who didn't receive the tailored dietary intervention (+26 g/day FV increase) [35]. Eight BCTs were identifiable from this RCT in total, including information-giving strategies regarding current dietary recommendations and health consequences of poor diet, problem-solving, action planning and tailored feedback based upon participants' dietary self-monitoring (from food diaries and a self-reported diet questionnaire). These findings illustrate a pattern of BCTs of importance identified from previous reviews [30, 32]. Despite limited follow-up in this RCT (6 weeks), the levels of additional FV intake reported in this trial may confer clinically significant improvements to health [4].

8.4 Integrating Behaviour Change Principles into Everyday Clinical Practice

In England, the National Institute for Health and Care Excellence (NICE) provides national guidance and advice to improve health and social care which is adopted by most of the United Kingdom. They produce regularly checked and updated Public Health Guidance on behaviour change (individual approaches published in 2014 (PH49) and principles for effective interventions published in 2007 (PH6)) [36, 37]. The most recent guidance outlines evidence-based strategies for behaviour change interventions in adults over 16 years across a range of health-damaging behaviours, such as smoking, poor diet and alcohol misuse, and is intended to be used by health professionals, commissioners and healthcare providers as well as the wider public. The guidance provides a number of recommendations to support individuals with health-promoting behaviour change, ranging from development of a local behaviour change policy and strategy, to planning, implementing and reviewing behaviour change interventions that meet local needs and ensuring that healthcare staff have adequate training in the principles of behaviour change. One recommendation specifically relates to the use of 'proven' BCTs, which are outlined specifically as 'goals and planning', 'feedback and monitoring' and 'social support'—all BCTs which have been consistently highlighted in successful dietary behaviour change interventions in this chapter.

Core public health guidance such as this which has been rigorously developed based on the available scientific evidence is particularly useful as it sends a unified message and calls upon the skills of multiple healthcare staff/professionals working across many levels of healthcare services. Embedding behaviour change skills and 'healthy' conversations into routine healthcare practice also aligns with 'Making Every Contact Count' (MECC), an approach used by both the National Health Service in the United Kingdom and the Health Service Executive in the Republic of Ireland. MECC enables the 'opportunistic delivery of consistent and concise healthy lifestyle information and enables individuals to engage in conversations about their health at scale across organisations and populations' [38]. Training of healthcare staff to understand the principles of behaviour change and effective BCTs is therefore vital to maximize the chances of supporting positive behaviour change in service users. One such approach to upskilling those working in government and policy through to frontline healthcare services in behaviour change is that of the Behaviour Change Wheel (BCW) [39]. The BCW is an evidence-based method for developing interventions (and policies) to change behaviour through a series of clearly laid out steps. At the core of the BCW lies the COM-B Model, which suggests that Behaviour (B) is the result of a combination of interacting factors: Capability (C), Opportunity (O) and Motivation (M) [39]. The BCW has been used to address issues relating to dietary behaviour change in adults, amongst many other varied behaviour change interventions and as such, the BCW should be considered a useful tool for anyone setting out to design and implement a behaviour change intervention [40].

8.5 Promoting Long-Term Dietary Behaviour Change

Presently, much of the available evidence on interventions for health-promoting behaviour change shows promise, in the short term at least (i.e. less than 6 months) [41]. However, long-term behaviour change, or behaviour change maintenance, is considerably more challenging [42]. This can be partly attributed to both a lack of long-term follow-up included within research studies and intervention effects diminishing over time [43]. A review conducted by Kwasnicka et al. highlighted a number of theoretical explanations of behaviour change maintenance which included the role of habits, alongside motives, self-regulation, psychological and physical resources, and environmental and social influences [42].

8.5.1 Habits

Habits have drawn particular attention in relation to health behaviour change strategies due to their 'automatic' characteristics. Habits are referred to as behaviours that have become automatically triggered through repetition of a given behaviour in a consistent context, suggesting that, once developed, they require minimal deliberation or planning and can be enacted without conscious intention [44, 45]. This suggests that once a person has developed a 'habit' for a certain behaviour, it should be more readily enacted as the

Table 8.2 Tips for making healthy habits (adapted from Gardner et al. 2012) [53]

Tool for patients:

Make a new healthy habit

1. Decide on a goal that you would like to achieve for your health.

2. Choose a simple action that will get you towards your goal which you can do on a daily basis.

3. Plan when and where you will do your chosen action. Be consistent: Choose a time and place (i.e.trigger) that you encounter every day of the week.

4. Every time you encounter that time and place (i.e. trigger), do the action.

5. It will get easier with time, and within 10 weeks you should find that you are prompted to carry out the action automatically when you encounter the trigger, without even having to think about it.

6. Congratulations, you have made a healthy habit!

My goal (e.g. 'to eat more fruits and vegetables') ____

My plan/action (e.g. 'after I have lunch at home I will have a piece of fruit')

(When and where) ________________________ I will ________________________

Consider using a tick sheet to monitor your progress in the early phases of trying to adopt a new habit—tick each day (Mon–Sun) when you manage to carry out the action you are trying to make habitual.

individual will experience an unconscious impulse to perform that behaviour upon encountering its specific cue or context. For example, if a person chose to have fruit with breakfast each day, after a sufficient period of repetition, merely encountering the cue—i.e. 'breakfast'—would elicit an unconscious impulse to include fruit as part of this meal, thus making healthy choices easier. Once developed, habits are considered to have acquired 'automaticity'—a measure of habit strength—whereby habits then self-perpetuate, as they are elicited upon each encounter of the cue or context, reinforcing the link between the situation and the behaviour [46–49].

Habit formation advice, paired with small, achievable dietary changes, has been tested as a behaviour change strategy across a number of studies to date [50–52]. In line with principles of MECC and promoting positive behaviour change in individuals/service users across multiple health service settings, there have been calls to embed habit-formation principles into patient interactions. Simple advice on how to make healthy actions into habits, i.e. externally triggered automatic responses to frequently encountered cues or contexts, could be a useful addition in the behaviour change toolkit, rather than relying solely on information and advice-giving strategies which rely on an individual's motivation, which typically wanes [53]. In lay terms, this means offering a patient advice on repeating a (healthy) behaviour consistently in the same context, for example,

having a banana with breakfast each day, until it becomes second nature [49]. An article on how to make health habitual in the British Journal of General Practice by Gardner and colleagues (2012) offers some practical advice on how health professionals might encourage habit formation in patients, even within brief encounters (see Table 8.2). Patients should be encouraged to choose their own new action (behaviour) to try and make habitual and to choose small and achievable changes. Furthermore, it is important to reassure patients that habit formation takes time (up to 10 weeks), and that the new action (i.e. healthy behaviour) should become progressively easier to carry out as it becomes a 'habit' [53].

8.6 Conclusion

Whilst it is clear that we need simple and sustainable dietary behaviour change which individuals can maintain in order to promote healthy ageing in spite of a changing oral health environment, there is promise for successful dietary intervention based on the current evidence. Advances in behavioural science have allowed for better descriptions and testing of effective strategies or techniques for promoting dietary behaviour change with the development of BCT taxonomies and the BCW. A number of BCTs relating to self-regulatory behaviours such as goal-setting and self-monitoring have shown particular promise with regard to dietary interventions in adults, across a range of population groups. Regarding long-term behaviour change maintenance, habits have shown promise by creating healthy behaviours which are automatically cued via context-dependent repetition, making the healthy choice easier in the long term.

References

1. World Health Organization. Healthy diet Factsheet. Geneva, Switzerland: World Health Organization; 2018.
2. Public Health England. National Diet and Nutrition Survey Results from Years 9 to 11 (combined) of the Rolling Programme (2016/2017 to 2018/2019). England, UK: Public Health England.
3. National Health Service. NHS Eatwell Guide. The Eatwell Guide: Public Health England in association with the Welsh government, Food Standards Scotland and the Food Standards Agency in Northern Ireland. Source: https://www.nhs.uk/live-well/eat-well/the-eatwell-guide/.
4. Wang X, Ouyang Y, Liu J, et al. Fruit and vegetable consumption and mortality from all causes, cardiovascular disease, and cancer: systematic review and dose-response meta-analysis of prospective cohort studies. BMJ Br Med J. 2014;349:g4490. https://doi.org/10.1136/bmj.g4490.
5. Reynolds A, Mann J, Cummings J, Winter N, Mete E, Te Morenga L. Carbohydrate quality and human health: a series of systematic reviews and meta-analyses. Lancet. 2019;393(10170):434–45. https://doi.org/10.1016/S0140-6736(18)31809-9.
6. Butland B, Jebb S, Kopelman P, McPherson K, Thomas S, Mardell JPV. Foresight. Tackling obesities: future choices. Project report.
7. Bray GA, Kim KK, Wilding JPH, World Obesity Federation. Obesity: a chronic relapsing progressive disease process. A position statement of the World Obesity Federation. Obes Rev. 2017;18(7):715–23.
8. Kleinert S, Horton R. Obesity needs to be put into a much wider context. Lancet. 2019;393(10173):724–6. https://doi.org/10.1016/S0140-6736(18)33192-1.
9. Hruby A, Hu FB. The epidemiology of obesity: a big picture. Pharmaco Econ. 2015;33(7):673–89. https://doi.org/10.1007/s40273-014-0243-x.
10. Lotta LA, Mokrosiński J, Mendes de Oliveira E, et al. Human gain-of-function MC4R variants show signaling bias and protect against obesity. Cell. 2019;177(3):597–607. https://doi.org/10.1016/j.cell.2019.03.044.
11. O'Rahilly S, Farooqi IS. Genetics of obesity. Philos Trans R Soc Lond Ser B Biol Sci. 2006;361(1471):1095–105. https://doi.org/10.1098/rstb.2006.1850.
12. Public Health England. Adult obesity slideset. England, UK: Public Health England. Source: https://www.gov.uk/government/publications/adult-obesity-patterns-and-trends/patternsand-trends-in-adult-obesity-national-data.
13. Finegood DT, Merth TDN, Rutter H. Implications of the foresight obesity system map for solutions to childhood obesity. Obesity. 2010;18(S1):S13–6. https://doi.org/10.1038/oby.2009.426.
14. Kazemi S, Savabi G, Khazaei S, et al. Association between food intake and oral health in elderly: SEPAHAN systematic review no. 8. Dent Res J. 2011;8(Suppl 1):S15–20.
15. Krall E, Hayes C, Garcia R. How dentition status and masticatory function affect nutrient intake. J Am Dent Assoc. 1998;129(9):1261–9. https://doi.org/10.14219/jada.archive.1998.0423.
16. Brodeur J-M, Laurin D, Vallee R, Lachapelle D. Nutrient intake and gastrointestinal disorders related to masticatory performance in the edentulous elderly. J Prosthet Dent. 1993;70(5):468–73. https://doi.org/10.1016/0022-3913(93)90087-5.
17. Marcenes W, Steele JG, Sheiham A, Walls AWG. The relationship between dental status, food selection, nutrient intake, nutritional status, and body mass index in older people. Cad Saude Publica. 2003;19(3):809–16.
18. McKenna G, Allen PF, Flynn A, et al. Impact of tooth replacement strategies on the nutritional status of partially-dentate elders. Gerodontology. 2012;29(2):e883–90. https://doi.org/10.1111/j.1741-2358.2011.00579.x.
19. McKenna G, Allen PF, O'Mahony D, et al. Comparison of functionally orientated tooth replacement and removable partial dentures on the nutritional status of partially dentate older patients: a randomised controlled clinical trial. J Dent. 2014;42(6):653–9. https://doi.org/10.1016/j.jdent.2014.03.005.
20. McCrum LA, Watson S, McGowan L, et al. Development and feasibility of a tailored habit-based dietary intervention coupled with natural tooth replacement on the nutritional status of older patients. Pilot Feasibil Stud. 2020;6:120. https://doi.org/10.1186/s40814-020-00654-6.
21. Linden A, Roberts N. Disease management interventions: what's in the black box? Dis Manag. 2004;7(4):275–91. https://doi.org/10.1089/dis.2004.7.275.
22. Dombrowski SU, O'Carroll RE, Williams B. Form of delivery as a key 'active ingredient' in behaviour change interventions. Br J Health Psychol. 2016;21(4):733–40. https://doi.org/10.1111/bjhp.12203.
23. Craig P, Dieppe P, Macintyre S, Michie S, Nazareth I, Petticrew M. Developing and evaluating complex interventions: the new Medical Research Council guidance. BMJ. 2008;337:a1655. https://doi.org/10.1136/bmj.a1655.
24. Abraham C, Michie S. A taxonomy of behavior change techniques used in interventions. Health Psychol. 2008;27(3):379–87. https://doi.org/10.1037/0278-6133.27.3.379.

25. Michie S, Johnston M. Theories and techniques of behaviour change: developing a cumulative science of behaviour change. Health Psychol Rev. 2012;6(1):1–6. https://doi.org/10.1080/17437199.2012.654964.

26. Michie S, Ashford S, Sniehotta FF, Dombrowski SU, Bishop A, French DP. A refined taxonomy of behaviour change techniques to help people change their physical activity and healthy eating behaviours: the CALO-RE taxonomy. Psychol Health. 2011;26(11):1479–98. https://doi.org/10.1080/08870446.2010.540664.

27. Michie S, Abraham C, Whittington C, McAteer J, Gupta S. Effective techniques in healthy eating and physical activity interventions: a meta-regression. Health Psychol. 2009;28(6):690–701. https://doi.org/10.1037/a0016136.

28. Michie S, Richardson M, Johnston M, et al. The behavior change technique taxonomy (v1) of 93 hierarchically clustered techniques: building an international consensus for the reporting of behavior change interventions. Ann Behav Med. 2013;46(1):81–95.

29. Greaves CJ, Sheppard KE, Abraham C, et al. Systematic review of reviews of intervention components associated with increased effectiveness in dietary and physical activity interventions. BMC Public Health. 2011;11:119. https://doi.org/10.1186/1471-2458-11-119.

30. Lara J, Evans EH, O'Brien N, et al. Association of behaviour change techniques with effectiveness of dietary interventions among adults of retirement age: a systematic review and meta-analysis of randomised controlled trials. BMC Med. 2014;12(1):177. https://doi.org/10.1186/s12916-014-0177-3.

31. Michie S, Johnson BT, Johnston M. Advancing cumulative evidence on behaviour change techniques and interventions: a comment on Peters, de Bruin, and Crutzen. Health Psychol Rev. 2015;9(1):25–9. https://doi.org/10.1080/17437199.2014.912538.

32. Dombrowski SU, Sniehotta FF, Avenell A, Johnston M, MacLennan G, Araújo-Soares V. Identifying active ingredients in complex behavioural interventions for obese adults with obesity-related co-morbidities or additional risk factors for co-morbidities: a systematic review. Health Psychol Rev. 2012;6(1):7–32. https://doi.org/10.1080/17437199.2010.513298.

33. Carver C, Scheier M. Control theory: a useful conceptual framework for personality-social, clinical, and health psychology. Psychol Bull. 1982;92(1):111–35. https://doi.org/10.1037/0033-2909.92.1.111.

34. McGowan L, McCrum L-A, Watson S, et al. The impact of oral rehabilitation coupled with healthy dietary advice on the nutritional status of adults: a systematic review and meta-analysis. Crit Rev Food Sci Nutr. 2020;60(13):2127–47. https://doi.org/10.1080/10408398.2019.1630600.

35. Bradbury J, Thomason JM, Jepson NJA, Walls AWG, Allen PF, Moynihan PJ. Nutrition counselling increases fruit and vegetable intake in the edentulous. J Dent Res. 2006;85(5):463–8. https://doi.org/10.1177/154405910608500513.

36. National Institute for Health and Care Excellence. Behaviour change: general approaches [PH6]. London: National Institute for Health and Care Excellence.

37. National Institute for Health and Care Excellence. Behaviour change: individual approaches [PH49]. London: National Institute for Health and Care Excellence.

38. NHS Health Education England. Making Every Contact Count. Source: https://www.hee.nhs.uk/our-work/population-health/making-every-contact-count-mecc

39. Michie S, van Stralen MM, West R. The behaviour change wheel: a new method for characterising and designing behaviour change interventions. Implement Sci. 2011;6(1):1–12.

40. Public Health England. Achieving behaviour change: a guide for national government. Source: https://assets.publishing.service.gov.uk/government/uploads/system/uploads/attachment_data/file/933328/UFG_National_Guide_v04.00__1___1_.pdf.

41. Frost H, Campbell P, Maxwell M, et al. Effectiveness of motivational interviewing on adult behaviour change in health and social care settings: a systematic review of reviews. PLoS One. 2018;13(10):e0204890. https://doi.org/10.1371/journal.pone.0204890.

42. Kwasnicka D, Dombrowski SU, White M, Sniehotta F. Theoretical explanations for maintenance of behaviour change: a systematic review of behaviour theories. Health Psychol Rev. 2016;10(3):277–96. https://doi.org/10.1080/17437199.2016.1151372.

43. Dombrowski SU, Avenell A, Sniehott FF. Behavioural interventions for obese adults with additional risk factors for morbidity: systematic review of effects on behaviour, weight and disease risk factors. Obes Facts. 2010;3(6):377–96. https://doi.org/10.1159/000323076.

44. Wood W, Tam L, Witt MG. Changing circumstances, disrupting habits. J Pers Soc Psychol. 2005;88(6):918–33. https://doi.org/10.1037/0022-3514.88.6.918.

45. Neal DT, Wood W, Quinn JM. Habits—a repeat performance. Curr Dir Psychol Sci. 2006;15(4):198–202. https://doi.org/10.1111/j.1467-8721.2006.00435.x.

46. Verplanken B. Beyond frequency: habit as mental construct. Br J Soc Psychol. 2006;45(Pt 3):639–56. https://doi.org/10.1348/014466605X49122.

47. Lally P, van Jaarsveld CHM, Potts HWW, Wardle J. How are habits formed: modelling habit formation in the real world. Eur J Soc Psychol. 2010;40(6):998–1009. https://doi.org/10.1002/ejsp.674.

48. Gardner B. Habit as automaticity, not frequency. Eur Heal Psychol. 2012;14(2):32–6.

49. Lally P, Gardner B. Promoting habit formation. Health Psychol Rev. 2013;7(Sup 1):S137–58. https://doi.org/10.1080/17437199.2011.603640.

50. Beeken RJ, Leurent B, Vickerstaff V, et al. A brief intervention for weight control based on habit-formation theory delivered through primary care: results from a randomised controlled trial. Int J Obes. 2017;41(2):246–54. https://doi.org/10.1038/ijo.2016.206.

51. McGowan L, Cooke LJ, Gardner B, Beeken RJ, Croker H, Wardle J. Healthy feeding habits: efficacy results from a cluster-randomized, controlled exploratory trial of a novel, habit-based intervention with parents. Am J Clin Nutr. 2013;98(3):769–77. https://doi.org/10.3945/ajcn.112.052159.

52. Lally P, Chipperfield A, Wardle J. Healthy habits: efficacy of simple advice on weight control based on a habit-formation model. Int J Obes. 2008;32(4):700–7. https://doi.org/10.1038/sj.ijo.0803771.

53. Gardner B, Lally P, Wardle J. Making health habitual: the psychology of "habit-formation" and general practice. Br J Gen Pract. 2012;62(605):664–6. https://doi.org/10.3399/bjgp12X659466.